DID YOU KNOW...?

- A woman's risk of developing breast cancer in her lifetime is 1 in 8.

- About 50% of women who develop breast cnacer have no apparent risk factors for the disease other than being older.

- 25% of the 500,000 breast biopsies performed each year turn out to be cancerous.

- Tamoxifen has been used for more than twenty years in the treatment of breast cancer.

- In 1998, Tamoxifen was shown to reduce the risk of developing the disease.

tamoxifen

NEW HOPE IN THE FIGHT
AGAINST BREAST CANCER

JOHN F. KESSLER, M.D.
and GREG A. ANNUSSEK

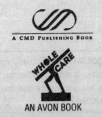

A CMD PUBLISHING BOOK

AN AVON BOOK

The ideas, procedures, and suggestions in this book are intended to supplement, not replace, the medical advice of a trained medical professional. All matters regarding your health require medical supervision. Consult your physician before adopting the suggestions in this book, as well as about any condition that may require diagnosis or medical attention. The authors and publisher disclaim any liability arising directly or indirectly from the use of this book.

AVON BOOKS, INC.
1350 Avenue of the Americas
New York, New York 10019

Copyright © 1999 by CMD Publishing, a division of Current Medical Directions, Inc.
Illustrations by Lydia V. Kibiuk
Published by arrangement with CMD Publishing, a division of Current Medical Directions, Inc.
Library of Congress Catalog Card Number: 98-91011
ISBN: 0-380-81028-X
www.avonbooks.com/wholecare

First Wholecare Printing: April 1999

AVON WHOLECARE TRADEMARK REG. U.S. PAT. OFF. AND IN OTHER COUNTRIES, MARCA xREGISTRADA, HECHO EN U.S.A.

Printed in the U.S.A.

WCD 10 9 8 7 6 5 4 3 2 1

CONTENTS

CONTENTS

ONE

WHAT IS BREAST CANCER?

QUICK FACT

A woman's risk of developing breast cancer in her lifetime is 1 in 8.

Susan, age 46, is a flight attendant who came to see me a few years ago after discovering a lump in her breast while showering. Susan was used to experiencing some lumpiness in her breasts shortly before a menstrual period, but this was something different. When the lump did not go away after several weeks she began to fear the worst and was worried that she had cancer. Fortunately, Susan's lump turned out to be a cyst (a fluid-filled cavity). I numbed her breast with a local anesthetic and used a very thin needle to drain the cyst and collapse it. Based on the color of the withdrawn fluid, I was very confident that the cyst did not contain cancerous cells. To be on the safe side, I had samples of the fluid sent to a cytopathologist for examination, who subsequently ruled out the possibility of cancer. (A cytopathologist is basically a pathologist who analyzes cell samples instead of larger samples of tissue.) Susan was clearly relieved by the news. Although her cyst required no further treatment, I told her that this was a good opportunity to become better informed about the health of her breasts, which she admitted she had always taken for granted. She had not had a mammogram (an x-ray of the breast) for several years and was not in the habit of examining her breasts. Susan was surprised to learn that about

50% of American women who develop breast cancer each year do not have any major risk factors for the disease.

Susan and I discussed the basics of breast anatomy and why the early detection of breast cancer should not be left to chance. I explained that most breast cancers originate in the milk ducts or lobules (milk-producing glands) of the breast, where they often remain for several years and pose no immediate threat. These in situ (noninvasive) cancers, as they are called, are almost 100% curable but are often so small that they cannot be detected by palpation (feel). High-tech procedures such as mammography—a procedure that uses low-dose radiation to create images of the inside of the breast—or other breast-imaging techniques are necessary in order to identify these cancers while they are confined to their original sites. (Even a palpable abnormality can be overlooked by someone who does not know the proper way to conduct a manual breast exam.) Once a tumor (a tumor is a mass of abnormal cells that may be either cancerous or benign) is large enough to cause symptoms, it has usually become invasive (penetrating)—breaking through the "wall" of the milk duct or lobule in which it grew and invading surrounding breast tissue. From there it can infiltrate larger portions of the breast and metastasize (spread) to vital organs or bones, which is a potentially life-threatening development. I gave Susan some literature on breast cancer including information on how to properly conduct a breast self-exam (BSE), which she had never done before. Susan walked away from what she referred to as her "breast-cancer scare" with a more informed attitude about the health of her breasts. She now gets mammograms and clinical breast exams every year like clockwork and feels less anxiety about her risk for the disease.

When tamoxifen (Nolvadex) was approved by the Food and Drug Administration (FDA) in 1998 as the first medication shown to reduce the likelihood of breast cancer in women at high risk for the disease, it was a historic moment in the history of cancer research. While tamoxifen has been used for years to help prevent the recurrence of breast cancer, the discovery of its role as a risk reducer in women free of the disease unlocked the full potential of this powerful medication. This exciting new tool in the fight against breast cancer is just one in a series of scientific advances in recent years that promises to dramatically improve the outlook of this often deadly disease. Improved mammography techniques and the widespread use of breast cancer screening have made it possible to detect cancers earlier, improving survival rates and increasing treatment options. Less invasive biopsy (the removal and analysis of a tissue sample) techniques, breast-sparing surgical procedures, and the increasing ability of doctors to predict the behavior of breast cancers by examining cellular traits also make it possible for women to have more choices about how to effectively combat their disease while minimizing its effect on their lives.

While these advances in breast cancer research are a cause for optimism, current statistics are a sobering reminder of how far we have to go. Excluding skin cancers, breast cancer remains the most common type of cancer in American women and the second most common cause of cancer death (lung cancer is ranked first). About 178,000 new cases of invasive breast cancer were diagnosed in American women in 1998, and almost 44,000 women will lose their fight with this disease in the same period of time. But statistics also reveal some positive trends. The incidence of breast cancer has leveled off in the last several years, and the number of women who die from the disease continues to decline due to early detection and more effective treatments. Between 1990 and 1994, the number of deaths due to breast cancer declined 5.6%, the steepest short-term drop in over 40 years. Overall, about 50% of women diagnosed with breast cancer can expect to be cured of their disease and live out the rest of their lives without recurrence, while for 33% the cancer ultimately will be fatal. A woman's lifetime risk of developing breast cancer is 1 in 8.

The progress made in the detection and treatment of breast cancer includes a new emphasis on the needs and preferences of the woman with breast cancer. Gone are the days when a breast cancer diagnosis automatically resulted in the removal of one or both breasts. But with empowerment comes responsibility. The fact that there are more options available today and that you have more power to make decisions about your care means that you must become an informed and active member of your health care team. Before you can assess whether or not to include tamoxifen as a part of the treatment or prevention program designed by you and your doctor, you must educate yourself about all aspects of the disease. This chapter explains what you need to know about the anatomy of the breast and the role played by hormones in breast health. The chapter also describes the general behavior of cancer cells and the specific kinds of cancers that affect the breast, and it outlines the factors that your doctor will seek to identify in order to develop a breast cancer profile. This profile can be used to predict the behavior of the disease and choose the best therapeutic options. See Chapter 2 for information on the causes of breast cancer and how to reduce your risk.

What does breast anatomy have to do with cancer?

Understanding basic breast anatomy is the starting point for learning how breast cancer develops and sometimes spreads to other parts of the body. The most visible characteristics of the breast—such as size, shape, position of the nipple, breast elevation, and color of the nipple and areola (the darker-hued, circular patch of skin that surrounds the nipple)—vary from woman to woman and do not appear to affect breast cancer risk. Your breasts are made mostly of fatty tissue and tough, connective tissue. In the rear portion of the breast, the connective tissue is attached to the pectoral muscles—the wall of muscle that separates the breast from the ribcage—and helps to support the breast against the chest wall. Contrary to what some women believe, the number of fat cells contained in the breast does not rise and fall in relation to changes in body weight. The number of fat cells remains approximately the same. It is the *size* of these cells that changes as your weight goes up and down. The reason your breasts get larger as you gain weight and smaller when you are slimmer is because the fat cells themselves are actually increasing or decreasing in size. Together, the fatty tissue and connective tissue surround, support, and cushion a milk production and delivery system. This system is composed of milk-producing glands called lobules and thin transport tubes called ducts. The

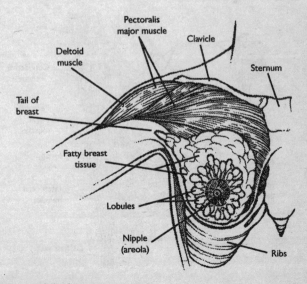

Anatomy of the breast.

ducts are designed to carry milk from the lobules to exit passages located in the nipple (called nipple pores).

How does this system of ducts and lobules actually work?

The system of ducts and lobules is a little more complex than the above description suggests. Beneath the skin, a number of ducts radiate outward from the nipple pores like the spokes of a wheel. Each of these ducts sprouts branches, on which are located the lobules. (Groups of lobules are referred to as lobes, and there are about 15 to 20 of these in each breast). Visually, the lobules are sometimes compared to clusters of grapes on a stem (the stem being the branch of a duct). Each lobule is composed of even smaller duct branches that bear tiny sacs called alveoli. The alveoli are the units within the lobules that actually produce and store milk.

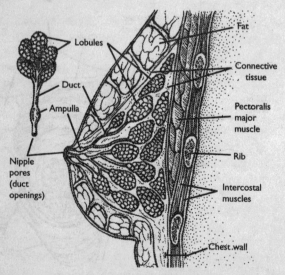

The system of ducts and lobules in the breast.

How is the milk propelled from the alveoli, the tiny milk producers, through the network of ducts towards the nipple? The answer involves the layer of tissue that surrounds each of the alveoli. This tissue, made up of myoepithelial cells, has the ability to contract and help expel the milk. The milk then travels through the ducts and into temporary holding areas called milk reservoirs (also called ampullae), which are actually just widened areas of ducts located near the nipple. Milk reservoirs are the last stop for breast milk before it is expelled through the nipple pores and into the mouth of a hungry infant. Tiny muscles contract during breast-feeding to make the nipple erect and to aid in the squeezing out of the milk being held in the milk reservoirs. As you will see later in this chapter, nearly all breast cancers originate in the ducts or lobules.

What are some other important things to know about the structure of the breast?

Your breasts also contain nerves, blood vessels, and lymph vessels. As most women know from experience, the breast has a rich supply of nerves, making the breasts very sensitive to pain, sexual stimuli, or changes in temperature. Painful breasts are not usually an indication of breast cancer but more commonly are associated with hormonal changes that accompany your menstrual periods. The job of blood vessels is to supply breast cells with nutrients and oxygen via capillaries (the smallest blood vessels). Lymph vessels resemble blood vessels in the sense that they are tiny tubes that branch into all the tissues in your body. But the work of the lymph vessels is different from that of blood vessels. Figuratively speaking, lymph vessels are the clean-up crew employed by your immune system. They collect the fluid that circulates between cells and sweep away bacteria, toxins, and cell debris to the lymph nodes, which are small filtering units (ranging in size from a pinhead to a bean) located in clusters in different parts of the body. Most

of the fluid collected by lymph vessels in the breast is filtered by axillary lymph nodes, which are located under the
arm (the medical term for the armpit is the axilla). Other
lymph nodes in the area are located in the chest and above
the collarbone. Lymph vessels and nodes are parts of the
lymphatic system, the system of organs and tissues that are
vital to your body's ability to fight infection and disease.
When breast cancer cells spread to parts of the body outside
the breast, they get there by traveling the highways of the
bloodstream or lymphatic system.

What do hormones like estrogen have to do with my breasts?

The hormones estrogen and progesterone are largely
responsible for the regular changes that occur in your
breasts with each menstrual cycle—lumpy breasts or breast
pain or tenderness—and for the more dramatic changes that
occur during pregnancy and breast-feeding and after menopause. Estrogen, the primary female sex hormone, is made
by the ovaries until menopause, when production ceases (a
small amount of estrogen is produced by other glands after
menopause). Progesterone is another important sex hormone made by the ovaries. Progesterone is closely involved
in your reproductive life and health and is primarily responsible for preparing the uterus for the fertilized egg and for
the growth of the fetus (developing baby). Estrogen and
other hormones function within a larger framework called
your endocrine system—a complex biological network
composed of organs and glands that secrete hormones to
other areas of the body in order to regulate reproduction and
growth, digestion, bone building, calorie burning, body
temperature, and metabolism. In women this network includes the ovaries, thyroid gland, pituitary gland, adrenal glands, pancreas, and hypothalamus. Think of estrogen
and other hormones as chemical message carriers. Once
produced by an organ or gland, they speed through the

bloodstream to specific receptors located on the cells of other organs or glands (a hormone fits into a cell receptor the way a key fits into a lock) where they either turn on or turn off—or speed up or slow down—activity at the site. Estrogen and progesterone are largely regulated by the pituitary gland in the brain, often called the master gland because of its role in a variety of endocrine functions. While certain levels of estrogen are necessary for good health, high levels of the hormone or a longer-than-usual exposure to estrogen have been associated with an increased risk of breast cancer. In some cases, estrogen also is thought to fuel the growth of existing breast cancer. For this reason, doctors usually investigate the estrogen-and-progesterone receptor status of breast cancer cells during a biopsy. If these cells are found to be "positive" for estrogen or progesterone, then one or both of these hormones may help the cancer to grow. If this is the case, hormone therapy such as tamoxifen may be used to put a chemical roadblock between the cancer cells and estrogen or other hormones.

What is cancer?

Cancer is the uncontrolled growth of abnormal cells, and it can affect just about any part of the body. Cells are the building blocks found in all the tissues of your body. The function of a cell and the way it behaves is governed by instructions it receives from genes located in the DNA of the cell nucleus. Normal, healthy cells in your body grow, divide, and die in an orderly, controlled process and are replaced by new cells with the same jobs and the same genetic instructions. Cells that die are replaced by new cells at approximately the same rate, so that cell turnover is more or less even. Cancerous cells arise due to changes in the genetic material of a cell. The result is a communication breakdown. Cancerous cells do not respond to the normal mechanisms that control the orderly birth and death of cells. With their genetic coding scrambled, cancerous cells run amok, continuing to grow and divide in an out-of-control fashion. They multiply more rapidly than normal cells and live longer but serve no useful purpose.

With cell turnover thrown out of balance, the longer-living cancer cells form masses called tumors. Tumors can invade and destroy healthy tissue and slip by the immune cell defenses designed to attack and destroy harmful invaders. A tumor can be confined to the site in which it originated or can metastasize via the bloodstream or the lymphatic channels. Metastasis occurs when cells from a tumor break away from the mass and spread—either regionally (within the same general area as the original site) or to distant parts of the body (for example, breast cancer may metastasize to the lungs or bones) where they form new colonies of destructive cells. As a rule, the further cancer progresses, the harder it is to contain or cure.

Who gets breast cancer?

While a small number of men develop breast cancer (1,600 cases a year, or roughly 1% of breast cancer cases), it is a disease that primarily affects women. In fact, being a woman is the single biggest risk factor—a risk factor in this context being anything that makes you more likely to develop the disease. About 77% of women diagnosed with breast cancer are over age 50, but this group actually has a better chance of surviving breast cancer than do younger women who develop the disease. Women who develop cancer when they are younger than age 45 have a 5-year survival rate of 79%, while women age 45 or over with the disease have a 5-year survival rate of 84% to 87%. How can this be explained? Doctors suspect that younger women have a poorer survival rate because their cancers are more aggressive and less responsive to hormonal therapies such as tamoxifen. It is not clear whether the poorer survival rate of younger women is related to the increased estrogen production of younger women or to other tumor-related factors. Incidence of breast cancer also varies according to race, ethnicity, and income. White women are slightly more at risk of developing the disease than are black women or women of other ethnic groups (although in women under age 50, blacks are actually more likely to develop the disease than are whites), while black women have lower 5-year survival rates than do white women. Women with low incomes who develop breast cancer are more likely to die from the disease than are women with higher incomes, because women near the poverty line often lack medical insurance or access to proper care and breast cancer screening. Breast cancer risk also varies with certain reproductive variables that are higher in women who deliver their first child at a later age and in those who begin menstruating at an early age or have a late menopause. At the current time there is no conclusive evidence linking breast cancer risk to the use of estrogen replacement therapy or to oral contraceptives. Hopefully these questions will be answered by future studies. Keep in mind that in order to create a risk profile for breast cancer, you must take many factors into account. See Chapter 2 for information on how to evaluate your risk.

What are the symptoms of breast cancer?

In the early stages of breast cancer, usually there are no symptoms. Most often, breast cancer is discovered as an abnormality on a mammogram before you or your doctor can feel it during an exam, a fact that emphasizes the importance of understanding your risk factors for breast cancer and having regular mammograms in order to detect the disease before it progresses. When symptoms do appear, they usually occur in the form of persistent changes in the breast such as a painless lump. In a small percentage of breast cancer cases (10%), there may be breast pain without a mass that you can feel. Other symptoms include swelling, thickening, skin irritation, discoloration, changes in the feel of the skin, or nipple discharge or tenderness. It is important to keep in mind that most changes that you notice in your breasts do not indicate breast cancer. More often they are associated with your menstrual cycle or signal the presence of a benign (noncancerous) condition. Nonetheless, if you notice any worrisome changes in your breasts, contact your doctor in order to determine what is causing those changes and to rule out cancer.

What are the most common types of breast cancer?

Nearly all breast cancers are carcinomas that originate in the ducts or lobules. A carcinoma is a type of cancer that arises in epithelial tissue, the tissue found on the surfaces of the body such as the skin or the internal linings of organs or glands. Carcinomas in a duct account for about 75% of cases, while those arising in lobules account for about 7% of cases. Breast cancer carcinomas can be in situ or invasive. The term in situ means "in position," indicating that the cancer is confined to its original site. In situ cancers account for about 15 to 20% of diagnosed breast cancers and have a more favorable prognosis than carcinomas that have spread. An invasive carcinoma is a cancer that has spread from its original site in a duct or lobule and invaded surrounding breast tissue and possibly lymphatic channels or blood vessels providing access to other parts of the body.

Are in situ carcinomas really considered cancer?

That is a good question. The short answer is this: For the purposes of classification, an in situ carcinoma (whether it occurs in a duct or lobule) is considered a form of breast cancer. But as you will see, doctors tend to view an in situ carcinoma as a precancerous condition if it originates in a duct and as a marker lesion for more invasive cancer if the carcinoma occurs in a lobule. What is the difference? Let us start out by discussing an in situ carcinoma that arises in a duct—termed ductal carcinoma in situ (DCIS). Also called noninvasive ductal carcinoma or intraductal carcinoma, DCIS accounts for up to 25 to 30% of breast cancers diagnosed each year and usually is discovered as an abnormality on a mammogram (more cases of DCIS are being detected these days due to the widespread use of screening mammography). Because it is an early form of disease, it rarely causes lumps that you or your doctor can feel during a manual breast exam.

The fact is that doctors do not know as much as they would like to about the natural history of DCIS because in the past it was nearly always treated with mastectomy, making it difficult to understand how the disease evolves in women whose breasts are intact. DCIS usually is unifocal (in one location) or multifocal (located in more than one position but still within a limited portion of the breast). The current thinking is that DCIS is a precancerous condition—what doctors call a direct precursor to invasive breast cancer. What this basically means is that if a case of DCIS is left untreated there is a significant risk that it will progress to invasive cancer at or near the site of the original DCIS. With less aggressive forms of DCIS, this risk may equal 30% at 10 years from diagnosis. More aggressive forms pose an even higher risk of invasive disease. See Chapter 4 for information on how DCIS and other types of breast cancer are treated.

Are some forms of DCIS more aggressive than others?

Yes. DCIS can appear as a variety of different-looking lesions and these lesions can be described by their pattern of growth as either comedo or noncomedo. The comedo type of DCIS has been identified as more likely than the noncomedo form (which actually includes a group of lesions described as clinging, solid, micropapillary, or cribriform) to progress to invasive disease. The comedo type is faster growing. It also is associated with telltale cellular traits—which can be discovered during a biopsy—that indicate a potentially aggressive cancer. These include an oncogene (a gene that contributes to the development of cancer) called HER2/*neu*. Cells of the high grade comedo form of DCIS often have extra copies (what doctors call "overexpression") of HER2/*neu*, which indicates aggressive cancer. These cells also tend to contain a mutation of a tumor suppressor gene (a gene that normally inhibits the growth of cancer) called p53, and this also tends to worsen the prognosis because the presence of this mutation is linked with cancers that spread.

What about an early form of breast cancer that develops in a lobule? Is that considered a precancerous condition, too?

No. Unlike DCIS, lobular carcinoma in situ (LCIS)—also called noninvasive lobular carcinoma—is not considered a direct precursor to invasive cancer and does not pose as great a threat as does DCIS. LCIS is considered a marker lesion—an indication that there is an increased risk of developing breast cancer in either breast at some point in the future. Women with LCIS have a 25 to 30% chance of developing breast cancer in either breast in the next 25 years. Interestingly, most cases of invasive cancer that develop after a diagnosis of LCIS are ductal cancers and only a minority are found in the lobules. (If LCIS were a precancerous condition, future invasive cancers would most likely occur in the lobules at or near the site of the original LCIS.) LCIS cells are slow growing, typically estrogen receptor positive, and rarely are associated with aggressive-cancer cellular traits such as overexpression of HER2/*neu*.

LCIS usually is discovered during a biopsy for a breast lesion that is thought to be benign. Women are diagnosed with LCIS at age 45 on average. The fact that LCIS is diagnosed more often in premenopausal rather than postmenopausal women may support the theory that LCIS tends

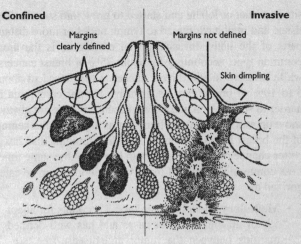

Confined

Margins clearly defined

Invasive

Margins not defined

Skin dimpling

Left: Lobular carcinoma in situ, (LCIS); right: cancer that has invaded surrounding breast tissue. In LCIS, the margins of the lobule are clearly defined; in the invasive cancer, the margins of the lobule are not clearly defined.

to regress on its own after menopause. Another explanation is that benign breast abnormalities that require biopsy are simply more frequent in premenopausal women. LCIS can be difficult to diagnose. Doctors sometimes mistake it for a benign condition such as atypical hyperplasia (an excessive growth of abnormal cells that increases your risk for breast cancer) or for the more serious DCIS. Getting a second opinion by having your biopsy slides examined by a pathologist (a doctor who conducts microscopic analysis of tissue samples) at another hospital is the best way to confirm your diagnosis. Unlike DCIS, LCIS is multicentric (located in more than one quadrant of the breast) in about 66% of cases and is found in both breasts about 30% of the time.

What about invasive types of breast cancer?

Invasive (also called infiltrating) ductal or lobular carcinoma describes a cancer that has spread from its original site in a duct or lobule and started to grow into surrounding tissue and may have spread to lymph nodes or more distant parts of the body. Invasive ductal carcinoma is the most common type, accounting for about 75% of breast cancers, while invasive lobular breast cancer is diagnosed in about 5 to 10% of breast cancers. Invasive lobular carcinoma is harder to spot on a mammogram because it does not always show up as a well-defined lump but as a general thickening of the breast instead. Invasive lobular carcinoma also has a better chance of appearing in both breasts at the same time. Less common subtypes of invasive carcinomas can be categorized as:

- **Medullary.** Medullary carcinoma accounts for about 5% of all breast cancer cases and has well-defined margins between the tumor and disease-free, surrounding breast tissue. Because of this margin, medullary carcinomas have a better prognosis than other types of invasive cancer.

- **Tubular.** As the name implies, this type resembles the tube-like shape of a duct. Tubular cancers, which account for about 2% of all breast cancers, are slow growing and rarely involve the lymph nodes when the cancer is small.

- **Mucinous.** A mucinous (also called colloid) tumor is a slow growing mass of mucus-producing cancer cells.

Are there rare types of breast cancer?

Inflammatory breast cancer and Paget's disease are rare forms of breast cancer. Inflammatory breast cancer, which accounts for 1% of all breast cancers, is an aggressive, quickly spreading carcinoma that causes the breast to appear red, warm, and swollen. The skin of a breast affected by inflammatory breast cancer also may feel thicker, appear pitted, or have ridges. This type of cancer occasionally is misdiagnosed as an infection and treated with antibiotics. Paget's disease, which also accounts for 1% of all breast cancers, affects the nipple and areola. Symptoms include a rash on the nipple or areola, nipple discharge, or an inverted nipple. Paget's disease usually is associated with an underlying carcinoma that is often noninvasive. Very rarely, a breast cancer may be a sarcoma (a tumor that arises in connective tissue or bone).

What determines my chances of beating breast cancer?

Prognosis (the outlook for recovery) is determined by a number of factors. The information gathered during biopsy and after initial surgery will be used to develop a profile of your breast cancer. This profile will be used to

---

Five-Year Survival Rates for Breast Cancer From Time of Diagnosis

As you can see from the statistics below, catching breast cancer early is the best way to improve your outlook for recovery.

- 92% when cancer is diagnosed at a local stage (confined to the breast). Only 60% of cancers are diagnosed at this stage, and regular mammography combined with regular clinical breast exams offer the best opportunity to increase this percentage.

- 87% when cancer is diagnosed at a regional stage (cancer has spread to surrounding tissue); 31% of cancers are diagnosed at this stage.

- 13% when cancer is diagnosed at a distant stage (cancer has metastasized); 6% of cancers are diagnosed at this stage.

Source: Adapted from American Cancer Society, Inc.'s Breast Cancer Facts & Figures 1997.

help determine your chances of recovery and the choice of treatments. The main features of this profile, which are discussed in more detail in Chapter 3, include the type of breast cancer, the site at which it developed, the aggressiveness of the tumor, whether or not the tumor has metastasized to lymph nodes or other parts of the body, and the receptivity of the cancer to hormonal therapy such as tamoxifen. Your age, menopausal status (whether or not you have completed menopause), weight, and overall health can also affect the prognosis and choice of treatment.

What are fibrocystic breast changes?

This is the term doctors use to describe the lumpiness or breast pain that most women experience during the 2 weeks or so before a menstrual period. These changes are perfectly natural and are not an indication of cancer or any other disease. As your menstrual period approaches, milk ducts and lobules can swell to form cysts (fluid-filled cavities) that put pressure on surrounding tissue, causing pain or discomfort. Almost always benign, these cysts can be microscopic or as large as golf balls—most are less than 1/4 in. in size. These cysts are usually soft to the touch, but occasionally they occur so deeply in the breast that they appear to be solid.

Fibrocystic changes tend to become more bothersome during perimenopause (the several years leading up to menopause) due to fluctuations in hormone levels. Most women enter perimenopause in their late 30s or early 40s. After menopause most women do not experience fibrocystic changes unless they are on some form of estrogen therapy, such as estrogen replacement therapy (ERT) or hormone replacement therapy (HRT)—a combination of estrogen and progesterone. The lumpiness or breast pain associated with one menstrual cycle usually disappears during the first 2 weeks of the following cycle. Any lump or other change in your breast that does not go away after a menstrual period should be looked at by your doctor in order to confirm the nature of the abnormality and rule out cancer. Your doctor will probably perform a fine needle aspiration (FNA) to draw fluid from the cyst and collapse it. In most cases, once a cyst is aspirated it requires no further treatment. See Chapter 3 for more information on how cysts are aspirated.

Is a fibroadenoma a type of cyst?

No, a fibroadenoma is a solid but benign lump. In fact, fibroadenomas are the most common type of solid, benign lump found in the breast. They can be as small as peas or (believe it or not) as large as oranges and usually strike women in their late teens or early 20s (they are more common in black women). Your doctor can confirm a fibroadenoma by doing a fine needle aspiration biopsy (FNAB) or a core needle biopsy. It is important to analyze tissue taken from a suspected fibroadenoma in order to confirm that the lump is truly benign and to determine if it harbors any abnormal cells that may put you at risk for breast cancer later in life. Rarely, a fibroadenoma may conceal a cancerous lesion beneath it. Depending on your particular case, you and your doctor may decide to leave a fibroadenoma

---

Rare, Benign Breast Conditions

In addition to fibrocystic changes and fibroadenomas, there are other, more rare benign conditions that may affect the breast. They may include the following:

- **Intraductal papilloma.** This small, warty growth occurring under the areola is difficult to palpate (feel) but may cause pain or a bloody discharge from the nipple.

- **Fat necrosis.** Usually forming at the site of a bruise or a surgical incision, a fat necrosis is a solid lump of damaged fatty tissue.

- **Duct ectasia.** This is a hard lump under the areola that results from a clogged milk duct. It is usually associated with nipple discharge and occurs most often in perimenopausal women.

in place or to have it removed in a procedure called an excisional biopsy. See Chapter 2 for more information on how certain benign breast conditions can increase your breast cancer risk and see Chapter 3 for more information on how a breast abnormality is biopsied.

TWO

KNOWING YOUR RISKS AND DETECTING BREAST CANCER EARLY

QUICK FACT

About 50% of women who develop breast cancer have no apparent risk factors for the disease besides being older.

Ann, age 57, is an entertainment lawyer who came to see me after she learned that her older sister had been diagnosed with breast cancer at the age of 63. Ann was concerned. She knew that having a sister with breast cancer greatly increases her own risk for the disease. I told Ann that by reviewing her medical history and lifestyle habits we could better assess her risk for breast cancer and discuss what steps she could take to remain cancer free. Besides having one first-degree relative (a mother, sister, or daughter) with breast cancer, Ann did not have any other significant risk factors besides being in a high-risk age group— over 30,000 women in the United States between the ages of 50 and 59 develop breast cancer each year. Ann was surprised to learn that being childless also increases her risk slightly. She wanted to know if the breast biopsy (the removal and analysis of a tissue sample) she had undergone 2 years earlier was a factor. I explained that, according to her medical file, the benign (noncancerous) mass removed from her breast at the time did not contain the presence of atypical hyperplasia—an excessive growth of abnormal cells that increases a woman's risk of breast cancer development.

21

Ann was relieved to hear that her just-completed mammogram (an x-ray of the breast) and the clinical breast exam I performed on her in my office did not reveal any abnormalities. Because Ann is at high risk of developing breast cancer in the future, we discussed how she could modify some of her lifestyle habits—such as reducing her alcohol intake—in order to reduce that risk. I was pleased to hear that Ann exercised regularly and ate a low-fat diet. I explained to her that by working out and maintaining a healthy weight, she can reduce her risk for breast cancer and for other diseases that tend to affect women in their postmenopausal years. Ann was interested in enrolling in an ongoing breast cancer prevention trial involving the medication tamoxifen (Nolvadex) that was being offered in her community. After examining the study protocol (the requirement for admission to the study) and finding that Ann had sufficient risk of breast cancer development to be included in the trial, I referred her to the medical center that was conducting it. Ann completed the study about a year ago and remains disease free today. I explained to Ann that while the potential benefits of using tamoxifen as a preemptive strike may prove to be significant, there is no hard proof that the protective effects of the medication last in the long run. I emphasized to her that it is still crucial to maintain a healthy lifestyle and be checked regularly for breast cancer. Annual mammograms and clinical breast exams in a woman her age are the best ways to detect the disease early when it can be treated very effectively.

———

While doctors do not know what causes breast cancer, they are beginning to zero in on the genetic basis of the disease and are continuing to enlarge their knowledge of the factors that may increase your risk. As you saw in Chapter 1, breast cancer occurs due to certain mutations (changes) in the DNA of a cell. These mutations render the cell unresponsive to the genetic mechanisms that control how cells grow and when they die, which results in destructive, out-of-control cell growth in a breast duct or lobule (milk-producing gland). Recent research has focused on two kinds of genes that appear to play key roles in the process by which a normal cell becomes cancerous: oncogenes and tumor suppressor genes. Oncogenes spur the growth of cells (in a healthy, controlled way), while tumor suppressor genes are designed to put the brakes on cell growth. Under normal circumstances, these two genes are vital to the regulation of orderly cell birth and death—your body's way of enforcing zero population growth among cells. But trouble can occur when flaws arise in either or both of these genes. An abnormal oncogene may become a superpowered cellular accelerator, fueling an excessive growth of cells, while a mutation in a tumor suppressor gene may render the gene unable to check the sort of uncontrolled cell growth that it is designed to stop.

A few years ago doctors made one of the most exciting discoveries in cancer genetics research—the identification of two tumor suppressor mutations associated with a vast increase in breast cancer risk for a woman who inherits either type of abnormal gene. But the discovery of these gene mutations only provides an intriguing piece of the puzzle. The number of women affected by these flawed genes is small. Most breast cancers arise from mutations in cells that occur during the course of a woman's life and are not inherited. While doctors cannot say with certainty what triggers the onset of breast cancer, they have identified a number of risk factors—a risk factor being anything that makes you more likely to develop the disease. Risk factors for breast cancer fall into two main groups: those you can and cannot change. They range from a family history of the disease to certain events in your reproductive life—such as starting menstruation early or experiencing menopause late in life—to health-related aspects of your lifestyle such as drinking alcohol or not getting enough exercise. These factors each present different degrees of risk, and in many cases doctors are unsure exactly how to define the threat posed by multiple risk factors. About 50% of women who develop breast cancer have no apparent risk factors for the disease besides being in a higher-risk age group.

It is important not to view your risk factors in isolation, but as a part of an overall program of healthy living. In some cases, caring for your breast health may coincide with your efforts to prevent other diseases. Maintaining a healthy weight, getting plenty of exercise, and limiting the amount of alcohol that you drink may not only help to prevent breast cancer but may also improve your overall health, cut your risk of developing heart disease or cancers that affect other parts of the body, and make you feel better in the bargain. More difficult decisions may arise when a risk factor for breast cancer provides potential benefits for other aspects of your health. For some women, the benefits of using estrogen therapy after menopause to strengthen bones and keep the heart healthy outweigh the small risk that it poses for the health of their breasts. Your doctor can help you put your risk factors into a proper perspective (most women tend to either overestimate or underestimate their risk) and craft a personal program of prevention that takes into account your needs and overall health goals. See Chapter 5 for information on how to determine if your high-risk status makes you a good candidate for tamoxifen (Nolvadex).

I'm a 28-year-old woman. Do I really need to be aware of the risk for breast cancer at my age?

Yes. While it is important to recognize the link between advancing age and the development of breast cancer (age is the single most important risk factor besides being a woman), age-related statistics can sometimes send the wrong message to younger women, who may take the health of their breasts for granted. It is true that 77% of women diagnosed with the disease are over age 50, and that women younger than age 30 account for only 0.6% of breast cancer cases. But by educating yourself about breast cancer now and evaluating your risk for the disease, you are in a great position to start taking steps—such as eliminating alcohol from your diet and getting more exercise—that may reduce your chance of getting breast cancer later in life. It also is wise to evaluate your risk factors at a young age in order to find out if you are in a high-risk group, especially considering the fact that in women at high risk, breast cancers often develop earlier and are more aggressive. If you are at high risk, you and your doctor can discuss the best ways to help prevent the onset of the disease or to detect it early.

Is it true that doctors have identified genes that cause breast cancer?

Cancer susceptibility genes is a better way to refer to them. You probably have read about the discovery of these genes—so-called cancer-causing genes tend to make

Age and Breast Cancer Risk in America (1997 Statistics)

Age	Number of women who developed breast cancer	Percentage of total breast cancer cases
29 or younger	600	0.6
30 to 39	8,600	4.8
40 to 49	32,600	18.1
50 to 59	33,000	18.3
60 to 69	36,600	20.3
70 to 79	43,500	24.2
80 or over	25,300	14.0
Total	**180,200**	**100**

Source: Adapted from American Cancer Society, Inc., Surveillance Research, 1997.

headlines—but these reports do not always separate fact from fiction. In the mid-1990s, researchers discovered mutations in two tumor suppressor genes—called BRCA1 and BRCA2—that greatly increase a woman's risk of developing breast cancer. If you carry a mutated form of either of these genes (which you may inherit from your mother or father), you may have an 85% chance of getting breast cancer in your lifetime. (These gene mutations are also associated with an increased risk of ovarian cancer.) It is important to understand that your body does not contain any genes that are *designed* to cause cancer. All of us carry some form of BRCA1 and BRCA2. In their normal form, these genes actually help to prevent onset of the disease by applying brakes to out-of-control cell growth. The trouble occurs when these genes become flawed and are unable to perform their jobs properly. To complicate things further, these genes do not always mutate in the same way. There may be hundreds of different BRCA1 and BRCA2 mutations, and some may present more of a risk than others. Breast cancers that develop from a mutation in BRCA1 or BRCA2 usually strike women earlier in life and are more likely to recur. Breast cancers arising from these abnormal genes account for about 33% of cases diagnosed in women before age 30 but are only responsible for 13% of breast cancers in women between the ages of 40 and 49. BRCA1 and BRCA2 mutations do not explain why so many women are affected by breast cancer each year. These genes only account for about 5 to 10% of all breast cancer cases in the United States.

How do I know if I have one these abnormal genes?

Your family medical history usually provides a clue as to whether or not you may have a BRCA1 or BRCA2 mutation. Such a mutation may be a possibility if you have more than three family members who developed breast cancer, especially if any of them developed the disease at an early age (under age 40) or had ovarian cancer as well. The number of Americans who carry one of these genes is relatively small—about 0.04 to 0.2% of the population. But certain ethnic groups may be much more likely to carry BRCA1 or BRCA2. For example, more than 2% of people of Ashkenazi (Eastern European) Jewish descent carry one of these gene mutations (that is about 1 in 50 Ashkenazi Jews), putting them at significant risk for breast cancer as a group. If you and your doctor suspect that you are a carrier of one of these genes, your doctor may recommend genetic counseling and a blood test to determine whether or not you are a carrier of BRCA1 of BRCA2. The purpose of genetic counseling is to explain the ramifications of testing and to help you interpret the test results. If you are found to be a carrier of one of these genes, you have several options. You may opt to have your breasts monitored more closely by having annual mammograms and clinical breast exams beginning at age 25 to 35 and doing a breast self-exam (BSE) every month starting at age 18 to 21. Some women may choose to have a prophylactic mastectomy (removal of one or both breasts before evidence of cancer is present in order to prevent the onset of the disease), while others may be candidates for the risk-reducing medication tamoxifen, though tamoxifen has not yet proven to be beneficial for women with these genes.

It is important to note that having a prophylactic mastectomy does not affect a woman's risk of getting ovarian cancer if she is a carrier of the BRAC1 gene, which is associated with a 45% lifetime risk of developing ovarian cancer. The BRAC2 gene, however, does not carry the same level of risk; it is associated with only a less than 5% lifetime risk for ovarian cancer.

If inherited cancer susceptibility genes like BRCA1 and BRCA2 are only responsible for a small number of breast cancers, why does the disease so often seem to run in families?

That is an important question. The fact is that most breast cancer risk associated with a family history of the disease has nothing to do with BRCA1 or BRCA2. Having a history of breast cancer in your family is a significant risk factor but usually does not pose the same degree of risk as do mutated forms of BRCA1 or BRCA2. For most women with breast cancer in their families, the risk of getting the disease does not exceed 30%. But this risk may increase depending on how closely related you are to a relative with the disease. If the relative is a first-degree relative (mother, sister, or daughter), your risk of getting breast cancer doubles. Having two first-degree relatives with the disease increases your risk by 5 times. As you saw in the introduction to this chapter, most cell mutations that give rise to breast cancer occur during the course of a woman's life and are not inherited directly. Women with a family history of breast cancer are more likely to have inherited a predisposition to certain breast cancer risk factors or to have adopted some of the unhealthy lifestyle choices of their parents.

For example, suppose that most of the women in your family experienced menopause later than age 50 (age 50 is the average). This may mean that you are genetically predisposed to go through menopause later in life as well. Because experiencing menopause late is an established risk factor for breast cancer (due to the fact that it increases your lifetime exposure to estrogen), you may be more at risk for the disease for this reason. There also appears to be a genetic component to obesity, another breast cancer risk factor. These are examples of what is meant by having a genetic predisposition to certain risk factors, and this predisposition is different from carrying an abnormal tumor suppressor gene that leads more directly to the development of cancer.

But the family environment in which you were raised can affect your risk as well. It is important to recognize that unhealthy lifestyle habits can be transmitted from parent to child in the absence of any genetic factors. If you were raised in a family that condoned the use of alcohol (particularly the excessive use of alcohol) or diminished the importance of exercise, you may be more likely to drink alcohol and exercise less as an adult. This concept of transmitting bad health habits from parent to child is not an entirely gloomy one. It creates the possibility that some portion of the risk associated with a family history of breast cancer may be minimized by adopting a more breast-healthy lifestyle as an adult and passing these values down to the younger women in your family.

What is the connection between estrogen and breast cancer?

Naturally occurring and synthetic forms of estrogen can affect your risk for breast cancer in a number of ways. The estrogen produced by your ovaries is vital to good health and has a number of beneficial effects such as keeping your heart healthy and building strong bones. But the fact is that the amount of estrogen that you are exposed to throughout life affects your risk for breast cancer because estrogen appears to fuel the growth of the disease. Your exposure to estrogen depends mainly on the timing of certain events in your reproductive life and on your use of synthetic estrogens (such as for contraception or as estrogen therapy after menopause).

- **Menstruation and menopause.** If you started menstruation early (before age 12) or experienced menopause at a late age (after age 50), this increases your lifetime exposure to estrogen and therefore slightly increases your risk for breast cancer.

- **Childbirth and breast-feeding.** Whether or not you have given birth to a child—and at what age—also affects your risk. Women who have had no children or who had their first child after age 30 have a slightly higher breast cancer risk. In fact, studies suggest that if you had your first child after age 30, you have a twofold to fivefold increase in risk compared to a woman who first gave birth before age 18 or 19! Breast-feeding may slightly reduce your risk for breast cancer (especially if you breast-fed for at least a year-and-a-half), but the evidence is inconclusive.

- **Abortion.** There has been some disagreement among doctors about the effects of abortion on breast cancer risk. Some studies suggest a link but others do not. A large study conducted in Denmark suggests that abortion is not a risk factor. There does not seem to be a connection between breast cancer and miscarriage either.

- **Oral contraceptives (the pill).** The use of oral contraceptives and its relation to breast cancer risk has been studied intensively for years, but the jury is still out on whether or not the pill poses any risk at all and, if so, how much. Most doctors believe that women who use oral contraceptives are at slightly increased risk of developing breast cancer while they continue to use the pill (this risk may rise the longer you continue to take it). But once you stop using the pill, the risk appears to fade: Studies suggest that women who stopped using the pill more than 10 years ago are not at increased risk.

- **Estrogen therapy.** The risk of breast cancer in postmenopausal women using supplemental estrogen has also been thoroughly investigated but, to the frustration of many women, the findings are not clear-cut. Estrogen replacement therapy (ERT) and hormone replacement therapy (HRT)—HRT is a combination of estrogen and progesterone—are given after menopause to reduce the risk of heart disease, strengthen bones, and help control menopausal symptoms. Most studies suggest that long-term use (for at least 10 years) of ERT or HRT is associated with a small increase in breast cancer risk. It may be possible, as one recent study suggests, that this risk exists only during current use of estrogen therapy, and that the risk may disappear once a woman stops using estrogen therapy for at least 5 years.

Can my personal medical history affect my risk for breast cancer?

A personal history of breast cancer and certain benign (noncancerous) breast conditions may increase your risk. For example, if you have had breast cancer, your risk for developing cancer in the opposite breast may increase by three or four times. This is not the same thing as a recurrence of breast cancer, which is discussed in Chapter 4. Having a previous case of breast cancer is considered a risk factor for the onset of new disease in the other breast. Benign breast conditions can also put you at increased risk, but it is important to make some distinctions here. Benign breast conditions fall into two main groups, proliferative and nonproliferative. Nonproliferative disease poses no increase in breast cancer risk. If you had a biopsy (the removal and analysis of a tissue sample) done for a breast condition that was determined to be proliferative without atypia (atypia indicates the presence of abnormal cells), you are at a small increased risk. Atypical hyperplasia (the excessive growth of abnormal cells) is associated with a greater relative risk of cancer development. Atypical hyperplasia combined with a family history of breast cancer increases your risk even more. Fortunately, most benign breast conditions are nonproliferative. In one study of 10,000 biopsies, 69% of women were diagnosed with nonproliferative conditions while only 3.6% were diagnosed with atypical hyperplasia. In addition to a personal history of breast cancer or benign breast disease, you may be at increased risk for breast cancer if you were ever treated with radiation therapy (in the chest area) for such diseases as Hodgkin's disease or non-Hodgkin's lymphoma.

Are there changes that I can start making today to help reduce my risk for breast cancer?

Eating right, getting plenty of exercise, and eliminating bad health habits are steps that you can begin taking immediately to lower your risk.

- **Maintain a healthy weight.** Being overweight appears to increase your risk of developing breast cancer, especially if you have completed menopause. Does it matter *when* you became overweight? It may. Being overweight since childhood and putting on weight later in life may present different degrees of risk. Some studies suggest that childhood obesity may increase the likelihood of adult morbidity (the relative incidence of disease), particularly with such conditions as cardiovascular disease and diabetes. However, an increased risk of breast cancer has been associated with excess weight gain later in life. More research may eventually shed light on this distinction.

- **Cut the fat.** The link between a high-fat diet and breast cancer risk has not been firmly established despite a number of studies. Some doctors believe that the type of fat that you eat is what primarily affects your risk for the disease. According to this view, monounsaturated fat—found in olive, canola, and peanut oils and in avocados—may actually reduce your chances of getting breast cancer, while polyunsaturated and saturated fat may increase your risk. Polyunsaturated fat is found in safflower, sunflower, and sesame seeds, soybeans and corn, certain nuts, and in the oils made from these. Saturated fat is found in high amounts in many of our favorite foods. Foods that contain large amounts of saturated fat include beef, pork, veal, poultry, butter, cream, milk, cheese, and other dairy products made from whole milk. Coconut oil, palm kernel oil, and palm oil—also known as tropical oils—and cocoa butter also contain high amount of saturated fat. The hydro-genated fat (fat that has undergone a process that causes it to become more saturated) found in many margarine products and in some prepared foods also may increase your risk.

- **Do not drink alcohol.** Drinking alcohol has been shown to increase breast cancer risk (perhaps by increasing estrogen levels). The more you drink, the greater the risk. Women who drink one glass of alcohol a day, for example, have only a small increase in risk, but that risk increases in women who have two to five drinks every day. You may be thinking, "But doesn't alcohol help to protect against heart disease?" While studies show that the incidence of heart disease is lower in women who drink moderate amounts of alcohol (one drink a day), most doctors are hesitant to recommend the use of alcohol for this purpose. This is mainly because excessive drinking is related to so many serious health problems, such as alcoholism, obesity, high blood pressure, liver disease, and stroke. Eating a low-fat diet and getting regular exercise are still the best ways to fight heart disease.

- **Quit smoking.** Smoking is a risk factor for many cancers (including lung cancer) and for heart disease, but as of yet there is no evidence that it contributes to the development of breast cancer. Many doctors expect to find a connection in the near future. Meanwhile, quit smoking for all the reasons we know about so far! Ask your doctor about the latest smoking cessation techniques.

- **Exercise.** Some studies suggest that rigorous exercise at a young age may offer lifelong protection against breast cancer. But just because you are a mother or grandmother does not mean that it is too late to enjoy the protective effects offered by exercise.

Even moderate exercise in adulthood can make a positive difference in your health. Exercise also is an effective stress buster and may improve your mood. Doctors suspect that exercise may lower breast cancer risk by reducing estrogen levels.

- **Avoid environmental toxins.** Some doctors believe that pesticides may be a contributing factor in the development of breast cancer. Once again, the connection relates to estrogen. Apparently pesticides may mimic the effects of this hormone—in effect,

---

Breast Cancer Risk Factors

Factors that you cannot change:
- Gender
- Genetic risk factors such as mutated forms of BRCA1 or BRCA2
- Age
- Race
- Family history of breast cancer
- Personal history of breast cancer
- Menstruation before age 12
- Menopause after age 50
- Personal history of benign proliferative breast disease
- Previous breast irradiation

Factors that you can change:
- Use of oral contraceptives
- Use of estrogen therapy (ERT or HRT)
- Not having children or having children after age 30
- Alcohol intake
- Being overweight
- Lack of exercise
- Exposure to environmental pollutants such as pesticides

---

increasing your exposure to estrogen. If you wish to avoid pesticides, switch to organically grown fruits and vegetables, available at your local health food market.

What is mammography and why is it so important?

Mammography is a noninvasive (nonpenetrating) procedure that uses low-dose radiation (x-rays) to create images of the inside of the breast. Screening mammography, which is used in women who do not have any symptoms of breast cancer, is the most powerful tool available in the detection of breast cancer. It has been shown to reduce breast cancer mortality in women age 50 or over by 30%. (Mammography is referred to as diagnostic when it is used to examine women who have symptoms of breast cancer.) Mammo-graphy can detect abnormalities in breast tissue that are too small or too widely distributed in the breast to be felt by you or your doctor during a manual breast exam. Mammography is capable of registering masses as small as 0.5 cm (about 1/5 of an inch). Due to technological advances, mammography uses less radiation than in the past (about ten times less than the amount of radiation associated with mammography procedures 20 years ago) and produces better images. As accurate as mammography has become in recent years, it is not flawless—about 10% of cancers are missed during mammography, partly because the breast tissue of younger women is denser and presents more of a challenge for the radiologist who interprets the images. Despite the effectiveness of screening mammography—and the fact that it has been shown to save a great number of lives—only about 50% of women who should have regular mammograms actually do.

What is the right age to start having screening mammograms?

That is an excellent question, and it is one that is a matter of debate even among experts at national health

How Do I Know if I'm Getting the Best Possible Mammogram?

The effectiveness of mammography depends on a number of factors, such as the quality of the mammography machine being used and the competence of the radiological technologists (who conduct the screening) and radiologists (doctors trained in the interpretation of x-ray and other images). Here are a few tips on getting the best mammogram possible.

- Choose a mammography facility that is accredited by the American College of Radiology (ACR) and the Food and Drug Administration (FDA). You can find an accredited facility in your area by contacting the American Cancer Society (ACS) or the National Cancer Institute (NCI). See Appendix A: Resources for contact information for these organizations.

- Make certain that the mammography machine being used at your facility is certified by the ACR. If it is, it will probably have a visible ACR seal on the surface of the device.

- Make certain that your radiologist is certified by the American Board of Radiology and that the radiological technologists conducting the screening are certified by the American Registry of Radiologic Technologists.

- Request that two radiologists examine your images to ensure the accuracy of the interpretation. If your facility does not do this, you can always have your images looked at by a radiologist at another hospital or facility. Ideally you should have a radiologist who specializes in mammography review your images.

- Do not wear deodorant during your mammogram. Deodorant can show up as spots on the images.

organizations. While the benefits of screening mammography in women age 50 or over are undisputed, doctors do not agree as to whether regular mammograms serve any useful purpose in women between the ages of 40 and 49. Mammography is less sensitive (translation: less effective at detecting abnormalities) when used to examine the breasts of women in their 40s or younger because these women have breast tissue that is denser and which can to some extent obscure the penetrating rays of a mammogram machine. Experts who are opposed to screening women younger than age 50 point to studies suggesting that screening women in this age group does not save lives. Their opponents believe that the potential value of regular mammography in women between the ages of 40 and 49 (who account for about 18% of all breast cancer cases) far outweighs the risk posed by exposure to radiation or the cost of these procedures. (Most doctors agree that the radiation exposure resulting from regular mammograms poses no significant health risk in women age 40 or over; the breast tissue of younger women may be more susceptible to the effects of radiation.) These same experts suggest that over time, follow-up studies may confirm more convincingly the lifesaving value of mammography screening in women under age 50. The NCI, ACS, and the ACR among other organizations recommend that women have regular mammograms (every 1 or 2 years depending on risk) between the ages of 40 and 49, and then have annual screenings starting at age 50. (Because the benefits of mammography in women between the ages of 40 and 49 have not been clearly established, many health plans only cover the cost of mammography in women age 50 or over.) For women at increased risk of breast cancer, most doctors agree that the benefits of starting mammography screening earlier outweigh the risks. Screening for breast cancer also involves BSEs and clinical breast exams.

What is the mammography procedure like and what will it reveal?

During a mammography procedure (mammograms cost somewhere between fifty to several hundred dollars and are usually covered by health insurance in women age 50 or over), your breast will be compressed between two plates in order to flatten and spread the tissue. Most women find this uncomfortable (not painful), but the compression lasts only a few seconds and it is necessary in order to get the best image. After the procedure, which takes about 15 or 20 minutes, a radiologist will interpret the black-and-white images of your breast tissue, which appear on a big sheet of film. An abnormality on a mammogram that suggests the possibility of cancer may appear as a starlike lesion; a small, irregularly shaped mass; or as a structural feature that looks out of the ordinary to the doctor's trained eye. In some cases the radiologist may identify white spots on the film. These are often microcalcifications (tiny calcium deposits within the breast tissue), which usually indicate a benign condition but are sometimes cancerous. Most abnormalities discovered on a mammogram turn out to be benign conditions such as a cyst or a fibroadenoma (a benign mass), but some are cancers. It is important to remember that a mammogram, while very good at detecting small abnormalities in breast tissue, does not indicate whether or not an abnormality is actually cancerous (it cannot even distinguish between a cyst and a solid lump). Only a biopsy can confirm a diagnosis of breast cancer. See Chapter 3 for more information on biopsy techniques and the diagnosing of breast cancer.

You may want to find out if free mammography screenings are available in your area. Breast Cancer Awareness Month (October) has resulted in the availability of free or discounted screenings that are sponsored by community hospitals or other health organizations on a limited basis. Check with your local hospital or clinic for information.

How to Detect Breast Cancer Early

The ACS guidelines for detecting breast cancer early are listed below. Following these guidelines is the best way to catch the disease early, when it can be treated most effectively.

- **Women between the ages of 20 and 39:** Monthly BSE and a clinical breast exam every 3 years.

- **Women age 40 or over:** Monthly BSE, annual clinical breast exam, and an annual mammogram.

Source: Adapted from American Cancer Society, Inc.

What is a manual breast exam?

There are two kinds of manual breast exams. A BSE is an exam that you perform on yourself or with the help of your partner. A clinical breast exam is done by a doctor or nurse trained to detect breast abnormalities by palpating (feeling) the breast. Guidelines for doing a BSE are designed to help you look for changes in your breasts in a more systematic fashion. By doing a proper BSE, you may be able to detect symptoms of breast cancer. These include a lump, breast pain, swelling, thickening, skin irritation, discoloration, changes in the feel of the skin, or nipple discharge or tenderness. By getting to know how your breasts usually look and feel, it will be easier to spot anything out of the ordinary. It is important to keep in mind that most changes that you notice in your breasts do not indicate breast cancer. More often they are associated with your menstrual cycle or signal the presence of a benign condition.

During a clinical breast exam, which is often conducted in conjunction with a screening mammogram, the examiner looks for some of the same abnormalities that you try to detect during a BSE. At the beginning of the exam, you will

Examining Your Breasts

By examining your breasts on a regular basis, you are more likely to notice any changes that occur. The best time to do a BSE is about a week after your period ends, when your breasts are not tender or swollen. If you are not having regular periods, do a BSE on the same day every month. If you notice any changes in your breasts, contact your doctor.

1. Lie down with a pillow under your right shoulder and place your right arm behind your head.

2. Use the finger pads of the three middle fingers on your left hand to feel for lumps in the right breast.

3. Press firmly enough to know how your breast feels. A firm ridge in the lower curve of each breast is normal. If you are not sure how hard to press, talk with your doctor or nurse.

4. Move around the breast in a circular, up-and-down line, or wedge pattern. Be sure to do it the same way every time, check the entire breast area (including under the nipple), and remember how your breast feels from month to month.

5. Repeat the exam on your left breast, using the finger pads of the right hand. (Move the pillow to under your left shoulder.)

6. Repeat the examination of both breasts while standing, with one arm behind your head. The upright position makes it easier to check the upper and outer part of the breasts (toward your armpit). This is where about 50% of breast cancers are found. You may want to do the standing part of the BSE while you are in the shower. Some breast changes can be felt more easily when your skin is wet and soapy.

7. For added safety, you can check your breasts for any dimpling of the skin, changes in the nipple, redness, or swelling while standing in front of a mirror right after your BSE each month.

Source: Adapted from American Cancer Society, Inc.

be asked to sit in a chair while the examiner looks at your breasts for any visible abnormalities. The examiner will use the pads of the fingers to examine the breast, usually in a circular motion. You may be asked to raise your hands over your head and push your palms together. This tightens the chest muscles and makes abnormalities more apparent. Later you will be asked to lie on your back and raise up each arm in turn. This is the more thorough part of the exam. Raising your arm allows the breast on that side of your body to flatten out, making it easier for the examiner to feel the deeper regions of the breast.

THREE

_____

DIAGNOSING BREAST CANCER: KNOWING YOUR BREAST CANCER PROFILE

QUICK FACT

Only 25% of the 500,000 breast biopsies performed each year turn out to be cancer.

Elaine, age 47, is a premenopausal aerobics instructor and a firm believer in early detection. Though not at high risk for breast cancer, Elaine never misses her annual mammogram (an x-ray of the breast) or clinical breast exam. Not too long ago during a screening mammogram an abnormality was discovered in Elaine's left breast. The radiologist (a doctor trained in the interpretation of x-ray and other images) identified the presence of microcalcifications (tiny calcium deposits that usually indicate a benign condition but are sometimes cancerous) that were multicentric (located in more than one quadrant of the breast). Microcalcifications such as those found in Elaine's breast are too tiny to palpate (feel) and can only be identified by sensitive imaging procedures such as mammography (a procedure that uses low-dose radiation to create images of the inside of the breast). Elaine and I discussed what the radiologist had found and decided to proceed with a mammography-guided needle biopsy (the removal and analysis

43

*of a tissue sample) to confirm whether the microcalcifica-
tions were harboring any cancerous cells. (Stereotactic
breast-imaging machines, which resemble mammography
equipment in some respects and take the same sort of x-ray
pictures, are also useful for a biopsy such as this but are not
available everywhere.) The pathologist (a doctor who conducts microscopic analysis of tissue samples) concluded
that Elaine had lobular carcinoma in situ (LCIS). I explained to Elaine that LCIS, while classified as a stage 0
breast cancer confined to the lobules (milk-producing
glands), is not a true cancer but rather a marker lesion—an
indication that there is an increased risk of developing an
invasive (penetrating) and therefore more serious form of
breast cancer in either breast at some point in the future.
Because LCIS can be difficult to diagnose—it is sometimes
mistaken for a benign (noncancerous) condition such as
atypical hyperplasia (an excessive growth of abnormal
cells) or for the more serious ductal carcinoma in situ
(DCIS)—Elaine's slides were examined by a second pathologist who confirmed the original diagnosis.*

*Elaine and I both felt confident that she had been diag-
nosed correctly. "Exactly how much risk are we talking
about?" Elaine wanted to know. I told her that a diagnosis
of LCIS meant that her risk of developing breast cancer
would increase by 1% a year for the rest of her life—for
example, around retirement age this additional risk would
equal about 20%. I also explained that doctors are unable
to reliably identify which cases of LCIS are more likely than
others to progress to invasive disease. We discussed the conventional approaches to managing LCIS. Elaine did not like
the idea of taking an uneasy, wait-and-see approach to
breast cancer development—in the form of annual mammography and a clinical breast exam about three times a
year in addition to monthly breast self-exams (BSEs). She
also felt very strongly that mastectomy was too drastic,
especially since she did not have any other significant risk*

factors for breast cancer. Elaine was interested in discussing the results of the Breast Cancer Prevention Trial, in which about 6% of the study participants had a history of LCIS. I told her that about 5 years of using tamoxifen (Nolvadex) was shown to reduce the risk of breast cancer development in women with LCIS by 56%. Elaine was impressed by the efficacy of the medication. After discussing the potential benefits and side effects of using tamoxifen as a risk reducer—including the increased likelihood of endometrial cancer (cancer of the lining of the uterus) and blood clots—Elaine opted to try the medication. She started on 20 mg of tamoxifen daily and after 2 years is still disease free. Careful monitoring of the breasts is also an integral part of her prevention plan.

It was only about 20 years ago that women were still living in what many doctors today would frankly admit were the dark ages of breast cancer biopsy (the removal and analysis of a tissue sample). The only available option in those days for women suspected of having breast cancer was a one-step procedure. Although the procedure was referred to as one step, it was actually composed of an on-the-spot biopsy followed by immediate surgical treatment and was carried out in its entirety while the woman was anesthetized on the operating table. In a typical one-step procedure, the doctor first removed a sample of tissue from the tumor (a mass of abnormal cells that may be either cancerous or benign) in the woman's breast by making an incision. This tissue sample was immediately examined by a pathologist (a doctor who conducts microscopic analysis of tissue samples) who was standing by in one of the hospital's labs. This analysis was also referred to as a frozen section examination because the tissue sample was rapidly frozen and then a slice of it was placed under the microscope for examination. If the sample was deemed cancerous by the pathologist, treatment was carried out immediately while the woman was still under anesthesia. This usually took the form of a mastectomy (the removal of one or both breasts)—a procedure the woman had preapproved ahead of time. This meant that a woman undergoing a one-step procedure did not find out for certain if she had been diagnosed with cancer or had lost her breast(s) until she had regained consciousness after the operation.

Today, thanks in part to the development of less invasive (penetrating) biopsy techniques such as needle biopsies, a woman with a lump or other abnormality in her breast has a variety of nonsurgical options available to help diagnose her condition. Most women diagnosed with breast cancer take several weeks to consider the best way to pursue their treatments. In this two-step procedure, as it is called, the biopsy is considered step one and treatment is step two. Before performing a biopsy your doctor will conduct a complete medical history and physical exam including a clinical breast exam (such as that described in Chapter 2), and may palpate (feel) the lymph nodes under your arm and above your collarbone for any indications that a breast cancer has spread to those regions. Your doctor will use images produced by mammography (a procedure that uses low-dose radiation to create images of the structure of the breast) or other imaging procedures to help detect and identify an abnormality, but only a biopsy can confirm whether or not you actually have breast cancer. Some of the most common types of biopsies are nonsurgical procedures performed in your doctor's office using a local anesthetic. A fine needle aspiration biopsy, for example, can be used to withdraw cell samples with a needle thinner than that typically used to draw blood. A core needle biopsy withdraws a cylinder of tissue about the size of a toothpick that can reveal almost as much about an abnormality as can certain surgical biopsies, some of which are quickly becoming obsolete.

Once a breast abnormality is discovered, the question to be addressed by you and your doctor should be, "What is the least invasive way to gather as much information as necessary about this condition?" The answer is not the same for every woman. The type of biopsy that you and your doctor choose depends on several factors, including the way the abnormality appears on an image created by mammography or other imaging procedures, its size and location in the breast, whether or not it can be palpated, whether you have a mass that appears in a single location or in clusters, and on your personal preferences. You should always ask your doctor to explain the various biopsy techniques, their advantages and disadvantages, and why your doctor recommends one over another in your particular case.

The amount of information gathered by the pathologist who examines your sample will depend to some extent on the type of biopsy you choose. The biopsy will reveal whether a problem is cancerous or benign (noncancerous) and whether a breast cancer is located in a milk duct or lobule (milk-producing gland). Breast biopsies also provide some indication of how fast the cancer is growing. The pathology report usually contains information about other characteristics of a breast cancer as well. As you and your doctor collect more information about your disease, you can begin to develop a profile of your breast cancer—a profile that will help determine the choices that you and your doctor make about treatment. Here are some important features of a pathology report (these will be discussed in more detail later in the chapter).

- **Type of cancer.** Your pathology report will indicate if your cancer is located in a duct or lobule and it may also indicate if your cancer is confined to the site in which it originated or has spread to nearby breast tissue. See Chapter 1 for more information on the types of breast cancer.

- **Tumor size.** The exact size of your tumor usually cannot be determined during a biopsy (except in the case of a surgical biopsy that removes the entire tumor) but can be estimated based on the image produced by mammography or other imaging procedures.

- **Tumor grade.** The pathologist will assign your breast cancer a grade (from 1 to 3) that indicates how aggressive the cancer appears to be.

- **Hormone receptor status.** This test will determine whether or not your breast cancer cells contain receptors for estrogen or other hormones. The presence of receptors indicates that these hormones may be fueling the cancer's growth.

- **DNA analysis.** What a pathologist discovers inside the nuclei of cancerous cells may affect the prognosis (outlook for recovery) for better or worse.

- **Genetic biomarkers.** The presence of abnormal HER-2/*neu* or p53 genes in your tissue sample may indicate a more aggressive cancer.

Is it possible to develop a complete profile of your breast cancer after your biopsy is complete? Usually not. A biopsy may provide many clues as to the nature and behavior of your cancer, but in most cases you and your doctor will not have a full picture of your disease until after you have undergone initial treatment, which usually involves some form of breast-conserving surgery or a mastectomy. It is usually after surgery for breast cancer that you find out the exact size of your tumor and whether the cancer has spread to lymph nodes or more distant sites. It is only at this point that a breast cancer can be accurately staged according to the TNM staging method, where T stands for tumor size, N for lymph node involvement, and M for metastasis (spreading) to more distant parts of the body such as the lungs or bones. Chest scans, bone scans, liver scans, and blood tests also may be ordered by your doctor during the course of your treatment to determine the extent of metastasis (if any). See Chapter 4 for more information on how breast cancer is staged.

What happens if my screening mammogram reveals some sort of abnormality?

The important thing is not to jump to any conclusions about your condition until your doctor has conducted further tests. While mammography is invaluable as a high-tech tool used in the front lines of breast cancer detection, more often than not an abnormality revealed by this procedure turns out to be a benign condition. The way a lump feels (if it is palpable), its location, and how it appears on a mammogram may provide your doctor with initial clues as to what the lump is and whether or not it is cancerous. If your doctor suspects that you have a cyst (a fluid-filled cavity), an imaging procedure called sonography may be used. Sonography uses high-frequency sound waves to create an image of the internal structure of the breast. It is more helpful than mammography in distinguishing between cysts (which are almost always benign) and solid masses (which may be either cancerous or benign). Unlike mammography, sonography does not emit radiation or cause any discomfort. In a sonography procedure, a hand-held instrument called a transducer (which looks something like a microphone) is moved over the breast containing the abnormality after a gel has been applied to the skin. While the transducer is moved, it sends sound waves into the breast tissue, which are bounced back and received by the transducer. The result is a sonogram (an image produced by sound waves) of the inside of the breast. This image appears on a monitor that looks like a television set.

How can I know for sure if my problem is just a cyst?

If your doctor suspects that the problem is a cyst based on how the abnormality feels or the way it appears on a sonogram, the next step is usually a fine needle aspiration (FNA). An FNA can be used to remove fluid from and collapse the cyst. Exactly how this procedure is done depends on whether the mass is palpable or not. If it is palpable, the procedure is relatively simple. After numbing your breast with a local anesthetic (this is not always required), your doctor will steady your breast with one hand while using the other to insert a very thin needle (thinner than a needle used to draw blood) through your skin and into the mass. If your doctor is able to withdraw fluid into the syringe, the cyst will collapse and in most cases no further treatment is required. To confirm that the cyst is benign, many doctors examine the color of the fluid taken from the cyst. Fluid that is clear or yellow is a very good indication that the cyst is benign. If the fluid looks bloody (which may signal cancer), it should be sent to a cytopathologist for testing. (A cytopathologist is basically a pathologist who analyzes cell samples instead of larger samples of tissue). If the sample is sent out to a lab, the results of testing are usually back in 1 or 2 days. If there is a cytopathologist on site at the facility in which your cyst was aspirated, you should have the results before you leave your doctor's office. If the suspected cyst is not palpable, sonography may be used as a guide to help your doctor locate and pierce the mass and attempt to withdraw fluid.

If my abnormality is not a cyst, can an FNA be used to get a biopsy sample?

Yes. FNA can be used to biopsy a solid mass but it is often not the method of choice. While it is definitely the least invasive type of biopsy procedure, in many cases a fine needle aspiration biopsy (FNAB) simply does not retrieve enough cells to provide accurate biopsy results. With an FNAB you run the risk that the syringe may withdraw normal cells and leave behind nearby cancerous cells, resulting in a mistaken diagnosis. But in some cases an FNAB can be an effective option. For example, if your doctor is confident from the outset that your abnormality is cancerous (based, perhaps, on its telltale appearance on a mammogram), it may make sense to perform an FNAB. In this scenario, your doctor will perform the biopsy not only to confirm whether or not your abnormality is cancerous, but to determine the nature of the cancerous growth. Several insertions may be necessary to get a sufficient sample for biopsy. As is the case with an FNA, sonography also may be used to guide the needle during an FNAB. If for some reason the FNAB retrieves no cancerous cells or if the sampling is deemed too small, you and your doctor can try a different type of biopsy procedure. An FNAB cannot distinguish cancer in situ (non-invasive cancer, or cancer that is confined to one area) from invasive cancer or certain types of abnormal cells. Core needle and surgical biopsies offer more information.

What if I have a mass that doesn't show up on sonography and my doctor is having trouble locating it by touch? Can my doctor still perform a FNAB?

Yes. As a rule, sonography is preferred because it does not use radiation—this is especially important for women who are pregnant. But there are cases in which a mass can only be seen on mammography. When this happens, a procedure called a stereotactic FNAB is used to help guide the needle into the abnormality in order to get a sample of cells from the area. Dedicated stereotactic imaging equipment (the word dedicated in this context means that the machine is *only* used for stereotactic breast imaging) resembles a mammography machine in some respects and takes the same sort of x-ray pictures. In order to get your breast into position for the stereotactic biopsy, you must lie face down on the biopsy table and place your breast through the opening in the table. Your breast (now on the underside of the table) is gently but firmly compressed between two plates.

Two x-ray images of the mass, taken at different angles, are then produced. These images make it possible for a computer to generate the three-dimensional coordinates necessary to zero in on the abnormality. The needle itself is held in a device called a biopsy gun, which is guided into position by the computer according to the coordinates. Your breast is numbed with a local anesthetic and the biopsy gun is placed against your breast. The needle is then injected into the breast and a sampling of cells is withdrawn.

What is a core needle biopsy?

A core needle biopsy is similar to an FNAB, except that the needle is thicker ($^1/_{16}$ in. in diameter and $^1/_2$ in. long). Because a core needle biopsy removes more tissue, it reveals more about the abnormality. More and more, doctors are relying on the core needle biopsy to get accurate information about a suspicious mass without resorting to more invasive surgical biopsies. During a core needle biopsy, the breast is numbed with a local anesthetic. The doctor then locates the lump by palpation and makes a nick in the skin in preparation for the insertion of the needle, which is held in a biopsy gun. When the needle has been inserted into the breast and is over the mass, the needle is projected into the mass and withdraws a core of tissue back into the needle with a clicking sound. Your doctor may tilt the gun at different angles and take several more samples without taking the needle out and reinserting it. After a core needle biopsy, a bandage is placed on the entry point. Complications are rare but there is a slight risk of infection. Any pain you may experience from the procedure after the anesthetic wears off should be minimal and can be treated with over-the-counter medications such as acetaminophen (Tylenol). If the mass is not palpable, sonography (as with a fine needle aspiration biopsy, sonography is preferred because it does not use radiation) or stereotactic breast

Why Get a Second Opinion of Your Biopsy Sample?

It is important to understand that the analysis of a biopsy sample is not an exact science. Your results depend largely on the competence and subjective judgment of your pathologist. Even top cytopathologists and pathologists may interpret the same biopsy specimen differently. When these discrepancies are minor they may not present much of a problem. But in other cases, misreading cells under a microscope can have more profound consequences. A ductal carcinoma in situ (DCIS), for example, is sometimes difficult to distinguish from a benign breast condition. If your pathologist misses the presence of DCIS, which carries a significant risk of a future invasive cancer, this mistake may put your mind at ease about the health of your breasts when you and your doctor should be closely monitoring them or weighing treatment options. Even when correctly identified, determining whether a case of DCIS is aggressive and how soon (if ever) it may lead to an invasive cancer is a tricky business even for experts. For reasons such as these, women are increasingly having their biopsy samples interpreted by a second pathologist, especially in cases in which DCIS is suspected or if there is any uncertainty about the diagnosis of a breast cancer or a benign condition—or even if a woman's common sense raises doubts about her initial pathologist's findings.

imaging may be used to guide the needle. The tissue removed during a core needle biopsy is examined by a pathologist. The analysis is usually complete in about 2 days.

My doctor has recommended that I have an incisional biopsy. I would prefer something a little less invasive. Do I have options?

You probably do. Without knowing the specifics of your case, it is impossible to debate the virtues of choosing this type of biopsy in regard to your breast cancer. But your instincts are correct to question the necessity of this type of procedure. While it is still performed occasionally for

---

Breast Cancer Biopsy Techniques

Nonsurgical biopsies

- **Fine needle aspiration biopsy (FNAB).** This technique is similar to a fine needle aspiration (FNA) except that an FNAB is used to withdraw cell samples for the purpose of analysis instead of being used simply to collapse a cyst.

- **Core needle biopsy.** The needle used for this procedure is thicker (it is $1/16$ in. in diameter and $1/2$ in. long) than that used for an FNAB. A core needle biopsy withdraws a cylinder of tissue about the width of a toothpick. Core needle biopsies reveal more information about a mass than do FNABs.

Surgical biopsies

- **Incisional biopsy.** This procedure, which involves removing a portion of a tumor by making an incision in the breast, has largely been replaced by less invasive needle biopsies.

- **Excisional biopsy.** This procedure involves the removal of an entire lump or mass. It is the most invasive type of biopsy procedure and provides the most information about a breast abnormality.

palpable lumps, the incisional biopsy has become something of a dinosaur among breast biopsy procedures. It has largely been replaced by less invasive needle biopsies. An incisional biopsy is an outpatient procedure that involves making an incision in the breast and removing a tissue sample from the tumor. The operation is done using local or general anesthesia. This procedure may leave a scar and, as with any surgical procedure, you run the risk of complications such as infection. You should always get a second opinion when your doctor recommends an incisional biopsy or any other surgical procedure. It would be a good idea to ask your doctor to explain why an incisional biopsy—as opposed to a core needle biopsy—is necessary in your case.

Are surgical biopsies totally outdated?

No. An excisional biopsy, which involves the removal of an entire lump or mass, is the most invasive type of biopsy procedure and provides the most information about a breast abnormality. While incisional biopsies have become a thing of the past—replaced by less invasive needle biopsies—excisional biopsies are still performed under certain circumstances to find out as much as possible about an abnormality. An excisional biopsy is sometimes performed when an abnormality is suspected to be benign based on the results of mammography, sonography, or an earlier needle biopsy. As you saw in Chapter 2, certain types of benign breast conditions may increase your risk of developing breast cancer. Removing a benign lump in its entirety, along with some surrounding tissue, may reduce the likelihood that it will become a site for the growth of cancerous cells in the future. Removing such a lump may also provide more detailed information about the nature of the abnormality— this information may be important in order to be aware of your risk for a future breast cancer. It is important not to confuse an excisional biopsy with a lumpectomy. A lumpectomy is a form of breast-conserving surgery used to treat an already diagnosed case of breast cancer. A lumpectomy may only be performed when there is a margin of cancer-free tissue around the lump. The purpose of an excisional biopsy is to find out what the abnormality is and to reduce any risk that it might pose to the health of your breasts by removing it. An excisional biopsy is performed in an outpatient facility or hospital. During the surgery, your doctor will make an incision in your breast and remove the entire lump. The incision will be closed using dissolvable stitches.

Removing a Lump that Cannot Be Felt: Wire Localization

In some cases, your doctor may recommend an excisional biopsy for a mass that is not palpable. This is usually the case when your mammogram reveals a cluster of microcalcifications (tiny calcium deposits that usually indicate a benign condition but are sometimes cancerous) or some other suspicious mass. In order to find out the exact nature of the abnormality, an excisional biopsy may be necessary. Because the area to be removed cannot be detected by palpation, the surgeon may need help in locating the abnormality. The solution is wire localization. Before surgery, your breast is numbed with a local anesthetic and a thin needle is guided into the mass using an image produced by mammography. Once the needle has entered the mass, a thin wire is inserted through the needle and into the mass. The wire has a hook on the end, which keeps it fixed in place. A second image may be taken of your breast to confirm that the wire is, in fact, anchored to the abnormality that is to be removed during the excision. Once this is done, the surgeon can proceed with the normal excision procedure, using the wire to find the exact location of the mass. The removed specimen can then be x-rayed to confirm that it contains the microcalcifications.

You may experience some soreness in your breast for a couple of days but it should not disrupt your normal activities. As with any surgical procedure, there is the risk of complications such as infection.

What is the significance of nuclear grading?

When breast cancer cells are examined by a pathologist they are assigned a grade (from 1 to 3), which is an important feature of a pathology report. The grade given to your breast cancer cells reflects their ability to divide and grow. Cancerous cells that more closely resemble healthy breast tissue are given a grade of 1. Breast cancers with a grade of 1 are considered to be slower-growing and less aggressive. Grade 3 breast cancers are faster-growing and more aggressive, and grade 2 cancers fall somewhere in between. Breast cancers with grades 1 through 3 are sometimes referred to as well-differentiated, moderately differentiated, and poorly differentiated, respectively.

Why do doctors check the estrogen receptor status of cancerous cells?

As you saw in Chapter 1, the hormones estrogen and progesterone are chemical message carriers. They help to regulate a variety of functions in the body by speeding through the bloodstream to specific receptors located on the cells of organs or glands (a hormone fits into a cell receptor the way a key fits into a lock) where they either turn on or turn off—or speed up or slow down—activity at the site. While estrogen and progesterone are vital to good health, doctors believe that these hormones may fuel the growth of certain breast cancers. For this reason, doctors usually investigate the estrogen and progesterone receptor status of breast cancer cells during a biopsy. If these cells are found to be "positive" for estrogen or progesterone, then one or both of these hormones may be helping the cancer to grow. If this is the case, hormone therapy such as tamoxifen (Nolvadex) may be used to put a chemical roadblock between the cancer cells and estrogen or other hormones. Women who have completed menopause are more likely to have breast cancers that are positive for estrogen or progesterone than are younger women.

What can DNA analysis reveal about my breast cancer?

Doctors can find clues to how aggressive your breast cancer may be by examining the DNA of the cancerous cells. Specifically, doctors examine what they call flow cytometry—the amount of genetic material in the cells and how fast it grows.

- **Ploidy.** Ploidy is the amount of genetic material in the nucleus of a cell. The other two key terms here are diploid and aneuploid. If there is a normal amount of genetic material in the nuclei of the cancer cells, they are referred to as diploid. If there is too much or too little genetic material in these cells, they are called aneuploid. Diploid cells indicate a more favorable prognosis than aneuploid cells, which indicate a more aggressive cancer. About 75% of breast cancers contain aneuploid cells.

- **S-phase fraction.** The S-phase fraction is a measurement of a tumor's growth rate and it is an important factor in the prognosis of a breast cancer. The S-phase fraction reflects the percentage of cancerous cells that are in the process of dividing. When it comes to S-phase fraction, lower is better. A lower number (such as 4) is considered favorable while a higher number (such as 15) indicates a more aggressive cancer.

What are genetic biomarkers?

Biomarkers are genetic characteristics of cancerous cells. They provide clues as to how the cancer will behave and these clues may influence how your cancer is treated.

They may even help doctors design new medications to fight cancer. Biomarkers are a relatively new and potentially powerful tool to help get a clear picture of your cancer and identify its characteristics. The most important biomarkers involve the HER-2/*neu* oncogene (a gene associated with the healthy, controlled growth of cells) and the p53 tumor suppressor gene (a gene associated with inhibiting the abnormal growth of cells). As you saw in Chapter 2, oncogenes and tumor suppressor genes are thought to be important in controlling (when they function normally) or contributing to (when they function abnormally) the development of cancer. Sometimes when doctors examine breast cancer they find what is called an overexpression of HER-2/*neu*—extra copies of the oncogene within the cancerous cells. It is believed that this overexpression of HER-2/*neu* helps to promote the growth of a tumor. This indicates a more aggressive cancer and one that may be less responsive to the effects of chemotherapy. Another biomarker that a pathologist sometimes finds in a biopsy sample is a mutation (change) in p53. Under normal circumstances, tumor suppressor genes like p53 put the brakes on the sort of out-of-control cell growth characteristic of cancer. But when a mutation occurs in p53, a cancer may grow faster. Many other breast cancer biomarkers are under investigation by researchers as well.

FOUR

SURGERY FOR BREAST CANCER

QUICK FACT

A lumpectomy followed by radiation therapy is as effective as a mastectomy for the treatment of early breast cancers.

Due to the widespread use of high-tech imaging procedures such as mammography (a procedure that uses low-dose radiation to create images of the inside of the breast), an increasing number of breast cancers are being detected in their earliest forms. Some of these cancers can be treated locally and do not require the use of adjuvant therapy (additional therapy used after primary treatment). Angela's experience with breast cancer illustrates how effective local therapy can be in the absence of additional medication. Angela, age 62, is a violinist in the city orchestra who was diagnosed several years ago with ductal carcinoma in situ (DCIS) that was unifocal (in one location). DCIS is an early, stage 0 breast cancer that is confined to the inside of a milk duct. It is difficult to palpate (feel) and usually is discovered as an abnormality on a mammogram (an x-ray of the breast). I had explained to Angela that DCIS is actually considered a precancerous condition—what doctors call a direct precursor to invasive (penetrating) breast cancer. If DCIS is left untreated, there is a significant risk that it will progress to invasive cancer by breaking through the "wall" of the duct in which it grew. This risk may reach 30% at 10 years from diagnosis. DCIS was treated with mastectomy (the removal of one or both breasts) so often in the past that doctors are still refining their knowledge of how the disease evolves in women whose breasts are intact. Fortunately, we know today that breast-conserving surgery accompanied by radiation therapy is as effective as mastectomy in a woman with early breast cancer (a cancer that is confined to the breast or that has metastasized only as far as the axillary lymph nodes).

Angela opted for a breast-conserving procedure and I concurred. Her cancerous tumor (a mass of abnormal cells that may be either cancerous or benign), which was about $1 \frac{1}{2}$ cm at its widest point, was removed via a lumpectomy operation along with a thin margin of surrounding, cancer-free tissue. Axillary dissection (a surgical procedure that involves the removal of the axillary lymph nodes adjacent to the affected breast in order to determine if a breast cancer has metastasized to the lymph nodes and how many are affected) was unnecessary because the risk of metastasis (spread) to the lymph nodes was so low. Angela's breast cancer profile indicated a favorable prognosis (the outlook for recovery). Angela had a noncomedo form of DCIS that was small in size and had a low grade (a number from 1 to 3, rating the ability of cancer cells to divide and grow, that helps to distinguish slower-growing from more aggressive tumors). The comedo type is considered to be faster growing and is associated with unfavorable cellular traits such as extra copies of the HER2/neu oncogene (a gene associated with the healthy, controlled growth of cells) and mutations (changes) in a tumor suppressor gene (a gene associated with inhibiting the abnormal growth of cells) called p53.

Angela and I discussed her prognostic factors and the potential benefits and risks of additional treatment. I explained to Angela that because her risk of recurrence or metastasis was a little below 10%, she did not require adju-

*vant therapy with tamoxifen (Nolvadex) or any other sys-
temic (whole body) medication. I was also concerned that
the use of tamoxifen might have increased her risk for a
potentially dangerous blood clot, which Angela was already
more likely to develop due to her hypertension (high blood
pressure). Angela received about 6 weeks of radiation therapy, designed to kill any remaining cancerous cells in her
breast or nearby tissues, which concluded her treatment. I
am pleased to report that Angela has kept all of her follow-
up appointments and remains cancer free. She is aware that
if her breast cancer returns it will probably be an invasive
and therefore more serious form of the disease. She also
understands that close monitoring of her breasts—in the
form of mammography, clinical breast exams, and breast
self-exams (BSEs)—is more important than ever.*

For decades, the initial treatment for most breast cancers
has been surgery to remove the cancerous tumor (a mass of
abnormal cells that may be either cancerous or benign).
While this continues to be true in the late 1990s, the types
of surgery used to eliminate cancer from the breast have
changed dramatically over the years. As you saw in Chapter
3, up until the late 1970s a diagnosis of breast cancer usually resulted in a mastectomy (the removal of one or both
breasts) that had been preapproved by the woman before
receiving a biopsy (the removal and analysis of a tissue
sample) under general anesthesia. The most common type
of mastectomy performed in those days was called a radical
mastectomy—the most extensive and disfiguring type of
breast cancer surgery. It involves not only the removal of the
entire breast and axillary (underarm) lymph nodes but also
the removal of the pectoral muscles that separate the breast
from the rib cage. This type of procedure has largely
become a thing of the past. Today a diagnosis of breast cancer no longer results in the automatic removal of one or both
breasts. While less extensive types of mastectomy are still

frequently performed in the United States, many women choose to have breast-conserving surgery instead, which involves removing a portion of the breast tissue while leaving the rest of the breast intact. Breast-conserving surgery, when combined with radiation therapy to kill any cancerous cells that remain in the breast, is one of the most important developments in the history of breast cancer treatment. Studies conducted over the last several years suggest that lumpectomy accompanied by radiation therapy is as effective as mastectomy (in terms of recurrence and survival rates) in women with early breast cancers—cancers that are confined to the breast or that have metastasized (spread) only as far as the axillary lymph nodes.

Once your breast cancer has been biopsied using one of the techniques described in Chapter 3, you and your doctor will have up to several weeks to analyze the report from the pathologist (a doctor who conducts microscopic analysis of tissue samples) and discuss your surgical options. A number of factors may determine the type of surgery that you choose. These include:

- The type of breast cancer
- Whether your cancer is in situ (in position, or noninvasive), meaning that it is confined to a milk duct or lobule (milk-producing gland)
- The size of the tumor
- Whether you have one or more tumors
- Whether you have microcalcifications (tiny calcium deposits that usually indicate a benign condition but are sometimes cancerous) that are multicentric (located in more than one quadrant of the breast)
- Your medical history or any medical conditions that you might have
- The size of your breasts

If you have an early form of breast cancer, you should ask your doctor if you are a good candidate for a lumpectomy or other form of breast-conserving surgery. You may be surprised to learn that some doctors do not always discuss these less invasive procedures with their patients, despite the fact that breast-conserving surgery has been shown to be as effective as mastectomy in cases of early breast cancer. Getting a second opinion regarding your breast cancer surgery will help you to make the most informed decision about your care. You should also ask your doctor for any literature on the type of surgery or other therapies that you are considering in order to educate yourself about your treatment options. Once you choose the type of surgery that you will have, it is important to discuss with your doctor how your breast will appear after the operation. Many women choose to have some form of reconstructive surgery after a mastectomy in order to help maintain their self-image or sense of well-being. Reconstructive surgery, which may involve saline implants or tissue taken from other parts of your body, can restore a more normal-looking appearance to the breast. It can be performed at the time of breast cancer surgery or years later. See Appendix A: Resources for more information on reconstructive breast surgery.

Initial surgery for breast cancer, which usually involves the removal of one or more axillary lymph nodes for analysis, is also used to gather more information in order to develop a more complete profile of your breast cancer—a profile that will help to refine your prognosis (outlook for recovery) and determine the course of further treatment. As you saw in Chapter 3, this profile begins to take shape after you receive a needle or excisional biopsy. After a mastectomy or breast-conserving surgery, the tumor and one or more lymph nodes will be examined by a pathologist. It is then that your breast cancer can be accurately staged according to the TNM system, where T = tumor size, N = lymph node involvement, and M = metastasis to other parts of the body such as the lungs or bones. (Tumor size and the extent of the axillary lymph node involvement are the most important factors used to determine prognosis in operable

breast cancer.) While the information gathered during an
initial biopsy can provide your doctor with important clues
as to how your breast cancer will behave and what sort of
treatment you will require, the staging of your cancer provides the most complete picture. How your breast cancer is
staged will help determine whether you will require further
treatment with systemic (whole body) therapy such as
chemotherapy or hormonal therapy. See Chapter 6 for information on chemotherapy and hormonal therapy.

What is breast-conserving surgery and why is it considered such an advance?

Breast-conserving (also called breast-sparing) surgery is
designed to remove a cancerous tumor while preserving as
much breast tissue as possible. Unlike a mastectomy, a
breast-conserving procedure does not involve the removal of the entire breast and usually requires follow-up radiation therapy. A number of procedures are considered to be
breast-conserving surgery, including a lumpectomy, quadrantectomy, and partial mastectomy. A lumpectomy involves removing the lump and a small margin (about a few
centimeters in width) of cancer-free tissue surrounding it.
This is the least invasive type of surgery for breast cancer
and preserves most of the breast. Other types of breast-conserving surgery remove more tissue. A quadrantectomy resembles a lumpectomy but it removes about 25% of the
affected breast, while a partial mastectomy is a procedure
that involves removing breast tissue. Breast-conserving
surgery is usually followed by about 6 weeks of radiation
therapy, which is designed to kill any cancerous cells that
may remain in the breast after surgery.

Many women with early breast cancers are candidates
for some form of breast-conserving surgery. Because these
cancers are being discovered at an early stage thanks to
screening mammography (a procedure that uses low-dose
radiation to create images of the inside of the breast), the
number of women who opt for these less invasive proce-

dures is growing. Breast-conserving surgery, for example, is sometimes used as an alternative to mastectomy in cases of ductal carcinoma in situ (DCIS), even when the cancer is multifocal (located in more than one position but still within a limited portion of the breast). (A carcinoma is a type of cancer that arises in the epithelial tissue found on the surfaces of the body such as the skin or the internal linings of organs or glands.) Breast-conserving surgery is not recommended if you have more than one tumor in your breast or have microcalcifications that are multicentric. Under these circumstances, it may not be possible to remove all the cancerous tissue and still preserve the breast as a whole. Pregnant women (first or second trimester) undergoing surgery for breast cancer are not candidates for breast-conserving surgery because the radiation therapy that follows may harm the fetus (developing baby). These less invasive surgical procedures are not options for women who have had previous irradiation of the chest area.

What happens during a lumpectomy procedure?

A lumpectomy is usually performed using a general anesthetic. This is necessary because breast-conserving surgeries such as a lumpectomy are usually accompanied by the removal of the axillary lymph nodes—the combination of these two procedures requires general anesthesia. During the lumpectomy procedure, your doctor will make an incision and remove the cancerous lump along with a margin of cancer-free tissue. The tumor itself and any lymph nodes that are removed will be sent to a pathologist for analysis. Where the incision is placed depends mainly on the location of the tumor within the breast. But within certain parameters you and your doctor may be able to choose a location for the incision that makes the resulting scar less noticeable after surgery. If the location of the scar concerns you, you should discuss the placement of the incision with your doctor well in advance of your operation. In some cases it is possible to position the incision so that the resulting scar cannot be seen even while wearing a bathing suit, night-gown, or revealing clothing.

If the tumor is located in the part of the breast near the armpit, your doctor may be able to remove the tumor and any necessary lymph nodes through one incision. Otherwise another incision will be made under the arm to remove the lymph nodes. The entire lumpectomy procedure, which may require admission to the hospital or be done on an out-patient basis, takes 2 to 3 hours. In some cases, doctors recommend an overnight stay in the hospital, especially if you have other medical conditions such as heart disease that may require close monitoring of your recovery from surgery. There may be some temporary swelling or tenderness in your breast after the surgery and the skin near the incision may feel hard due to the scar tissue that forms there.

If breast-conserving surgery is so effective, why are doctors performing so many mastectomies?

That is a very good question, and the answer is not entirely clear. A large study conducted jointly by the American College of Surgeons (ACS) and the American College of Radiology (ACR) helps to shed some light on why breast-conserving surgery is being underused. This study involved almost 18,000 American women with breast cancer (stage 1 or stage 2) being treated at hundreds of medical institutions in 1994. It studied patterns of breast cancer care and sought to determine some of the factors that doctors consider when selecting patients for breast-conserving surgery versus mastectomy. One of the first things that researchers noticed when analyzing the data from this study is that the overall percentage of women who received breast-conserving surgery was a relatively low 44%. Most experts believe that the number of women with breast cancer who are good candidates for breast-conserving surgery is higher. What is the magic number? No one knows for certain. The conventional thinking is that about 70% of breast cancer patients can be spared mastectomy in favor of less invasive procedures.

Why did so few of the women in this study undergo breast-conserving surgery?

The study identified a number of factors that appear to affect who gets breast-conserving surgery and who does not. As you have seen earlier in this chapter, breast-conserving surgery may be contraindicated (ruled out) for sound medical reasons such as multiple tumors, multicentric microcalcifications, previous irradiation to the chest, or pregnancy (first or second trimester). But this study suggests that many doctors in the United States are discouraging the use of breast-conserving surgery when prognostic factors (factors that affect the outlook for recovery) suggest that a cancer is likely to recur or metastasize. These factors include lymph node status, tumor size, and grade, which is a number from 1 to 3, rating the ability of cancer cells to divide and grow, that helps to distinguish slower-growing from more aggressive tumors. Some data from the study:

- About 53% of women with stage 1 cancers were treated with breast-conserving surgery as compared to 33% of women with stage 2 cancers (stage 2 cancers are either larger than stage 1 tumors or involve axillary lymph nodes or both).

- About 47% of women with node-negative cancers—cancers that have not metastasized to the axillary lymph nodes—received breast-conserving surgery while only 32% of women with node-positive cancers—cancers that have metastasized to the axillary lymph nodes—were treated with this kind of surgery.

- Women who had cancers with grades of 2 were 19% more likely to have mastectomies than women with grade 1 tumors (grade 2 indicates a more aggressive cancer than grade 1).

As you can see, these statistics suggest that in some cases doctors are using prognostic factors—such as the presence of a large tumor or one that has aggressive cellular features or has metastasized to the axillary lymph nodes—as major determinants when recommending mastectomy over breast-conserving surgery, even though these factors do not strictly contraindicate breast-conserving surgery. Aggressive cancers that threaten to recur or metastasize do not always justify mastectomy. In some of these cases mastectomy is unnecessary because breast-conserving surgery can be as effective as mastectomy in terms of recurrence and the risk of metastases is best reduced with systemic therapy and *not* the removal of the entire breast.

The study also suggests that breast-conserving surgery is sometimes discouraged based on age, health insurance concerns, and even geographic location. Older women are more likely to receive mastectomies than younger women—in fact, with each decade of life, the likelihood of undergoing a mastectomy increased 11% in the study. Women who were uninsured or receiving Medicaid were 19% (women with Medicare were 27%) more likely to have mastectomies than women with private health insurance or those in managed care plans. Perhaps the strangest statistic from the study relates to how the use of mastectomy varies according to regions of the country: Women living in the Northeast and Pacific Coast regions were about *40% less likely* to have mastectomies than those living in the Midwest.

What's the difference between one type of mastectomy and another?

As you saw earlier in this chapter, the most commonly performed mastectomy 20 years ago was called a radical mastectomy. This involves the removal of the entire breast, lymph nodes, and the pectoral muscles. This is the most

invasive and disfiguring type of mastectomy and compli-
cates any efforts to perform reconstructive surgery to
restore a more normal-looking appearance to the breast.
Over the last 2 decades the radical mastectomy has been
replaced by the modified radical mastectomy. This procedure is just as effective as its more invasive predecessor and
is now the most frequently performed breast cancer surgery
in the United States. In the modified radical mastectomy,
the breast is removed along with one or more lymph nodes
but the pectoral muscles are left in place. Another type of
mastectomy is called a simple mastectomy. It involves the
removal of the entire breast but no lymph nodes are taken
out. A simple mastectomy may be used, for example, to
treat a case of DCIS that cannot be treated with less invasive
breast-conserving surgery because the cancer occurs in too
many areas of the breast. Because all types of mastectomy
(except for a partial mastectomy) remove the entire breast,
radiation therapy is usually unnecessary.

What can I expect during a modified radical mas-
tectomy?

While you are under general anesthesia, your doctor will
make a large incision and remove all the breast tissue above
the pectoral muscles. This tissue reaches up to the collarbone and over to the armpit. Your doctor will use this same
incision to remove the lymph nodes. Some of this tissue and
any lymph nodes that are removed will be sent to a pathologist for analysis. The operation takes about 3 hours and
usually requires several days in the hospital, though some
mastectomies are now performed on an outpatient basis.
When you regain consciousness after the operation there
will be a dressing over the incision and probably a flexible
plastic tube emerging from it. This tube is there to drain the
fluid that can build up in the area of the incision. It is a temporary measure and will be removed after about 3 or 4 days.
As a result of this surgery you will have a long scar running
across the top of your chest that is roughly horizontal. The
nerves that serve the affected breast are cut during surgery,

so the area will be permanently numbed. You will probably have difficulty moving your arm immediately after surgery. This common side effect, which is different from lymphedema (see sidebar, below), will not last. Your doctor will show you exercises that you can begin doing 1 or 2 days

Types of Breast Cancer Surgery

Breast-conserving surgeries (these procedures are usually followed by about 6 weeks of radiation therapy)

- **Lumpectomy.** This procedure involves the removal of the tumor and a few centimeters of surrounding, cancer-free tissue. Lymph nodes may also be removed.

- **Quadrantectomy.** A quadrantectomy is similar to a lumpectomy except that it removes more tissue—about 25% of the breast. Lymph nodes may also be removed.

- **Partial mastectomy.** This surgery involves removing about 50% of breast tissue. Lymph nodes may also be removed.

Mastectomy (radiation therapy is usually unnecessary after a mastectomy)

- **Simple mastectomy.** A simple mastectomy involves the removal of the entire breast but the lymph nodes are left in place.

- **Modified radical mastectomy.** During this procedure, the entire breast is removed along with the lymph nodes. This is the most frequently performed breast cancer surgery in the United States.

- **Radical mastectomy.** This outdated procedure involves the removal of the entire breast, the pectoral muscles that lie behind it, and the lymph nodes.

after surgery in order to get your arm moving again. See Chapter 8 for information on the emotional consequences of a mastectomy and on reconstructive breast surgery.

What is an axillary dissection?

This is a surgical procedure that involves the removal of the axillary lymph nodes adjacent to the affected breast in order to determine if a breast cancer has metastasized to the lymph nodes and how many are affected. As you saw in Chapter 1, lymph nodes are small filtering units (ranging in size from a pinhead to a bean) located in clusters in different parts of the body. Tiny tubes called lymph vessels, which branch into all the tissues in your body, collect the fluid that circulates between cells and sweep away bacteria, toxins, and cell debris to the lymph nodes. Cancerous cells can also travel through these vessels to the lymph nodes and beyond. An axillary dissection is usually performed at the same time as breast-cancer surgery except in the case of a simple mastectomy or during breast-conserving surgery for an in situ cancer. Typically about 12 lymph nodes are removed during an axillary dissection, but that number may vary slightly from case to case. The lymph nodes are then sent to a pathologist for examination.

Doctors once believed that removing the axillary lymph nodes of a woman with breast cancer was therapeutic—that it could help prevent the cancer from metastasizing to other parts of the body such as the lungs or bones. But doctors no longer believe this to be true. Instead, they believe that systemic therapy such as chemotherapy or hormonal therapy is the most effective way to treat breast cancers that metastasize to other parts of the body. Axillary lymph nodes are removed and analyzed to help determine your risk for metastasis and your future treatment options. In the case of an in situ breast cancer, removing the lymph nodes is unnecessary because this type of cancer is, by definition, confined to the site in the milk duct or lobule (milk-producing gland) in which it originated. As you saw earlier in this chapter, during a lumpectomy your doctor may be able to remove the lymph nodes through the same incision used to take out the cancerous tumor if it is located in the upper part of the breast near the armpit. If the tumor is located elsewhere, your doctor will make a 2-in. incision near the bottom of your armpit in order to remove the lymph nodes, which are surrounded by fatty tissue. During a mastectomy, the lymph nodes are removed through the same incision that is used to remove the breast tissue. Complications associated with axillary dissection include lymphedema (see sidebar), permanent numbness of the underarm due to the severing of nerves there, and loss of shoulder mobility.

Is it true that there is now an alternative to having an axillary dissection?

This is true. A sentinel node biopsy is a new type of surgical procedure used to sample axillary lymph nodes for the

Lymphedema

The major risk associated with an axillary dissection is lymphedema—the swelling of the arm due to the buildup of lymphatic fluid that cannot drain in the absence of the lymph nodes. It occurs in about 10 to 20% of women who undergo the procedure. Lymphedema can occur immediately after surgery or years later. An injury or infection affecting the arm or hand on the affected side of the body may lead to the development of lymphedema or make it worse, so be sure to seek treatment for any injuries or breaks in the skin that may lead to infection. There is no cure for lymphedema but there are ways to manage it. If you suffer from lymphedema, your doctor may recommend physical therapy or a compression garment. Certain exercises may help the area to drain and alleviate swelling. The symptoms of lymphedema include swelling or tightness in the arm or hand.

presence of cancerous cells. It has two major advantages over an axillary dissection: It is less invasive and does not carry the risk of lymphedema. Unlike an axillary dissection, a sentinel node biopsy does not involve the removal of all the axillary lymph nodes adjacent to the affected breast in order to rule out the presence of cancerous cells. In this new procedure, the only lymph node initially removed is the one that first receives fluid from the lymph vessels (referred to as the sentinel node). If this lymph node is analyzed and found to be cancer free, there is an over 95% chance that nearby lymph nodes are cancer free as well—there is no need to remove them. In a sentinel node biopsy, a radioactive substance or a blue dye is injected into the area of the cancerous tumor. The radioactive substance or the dye is then transported through the lymph vessels to the sentinel node. A doctor can locate the sentinel node by spotting the presence of the dye visually or using a geiger counter to detect the location of the radioactive substance. Once this sentinel node is located, it is removed and examined by a pathologist. If it is found to harbor cancerous cells, more lymph nodes will be removed in order to determine how many are affected. As of now, the axillary dissection is the conventional way of determining lymph node status. But if studies continue to show the effectiveness of the sentinel node biopsy, this procedure may become the standard method of sampling axillary lymph nodes.

What is radiation therapy?

Radiation therapy, which typically uses a beam of radiation targeted at certain areas of the breast, is almost always recommended after a lumpectomy or other breast-conserving surgery to kill any cancerous cells that may remain in the breast or nearby tissues. (Radiation therapy can also be used before surgery to shrink a tumor.) Radiation therapy usually begins several weeks after initial surgery for breast cancer. While the radiation therapy methods of the past were effective in treating breast cancer, they were a little clumsy by today's standards. In the past, the technology

---

Most Important Factors Used to Assess Prognosis

- Number of cancerous axillary lymph nodes
- Tumor size
- TNM stage
- Tumor grade
- Estrogen and progesterone receptor status
- Ploidy (the amount of genetic material in the nucleus of a cell, which may determine how aggressive a cancer may be)
- S-phase fraction
- HER2/*neu* overexpression

---

needed to precisely target the radiation was not available. As a result, wayward radiation sometimes caused new cancers or other medical problems. Today, doctors can focus x-rays or gamma rays with a high degree of precision into the areas of the breast where doctors suspect there may be remaining cancer cells. Radiation therapy actually affects both normal and cancerous cells, but the normal cells recover while the cancerous cells die. As you saw earlier in this chapter, radiation therapy is not usually necessary after a mastectomy. But there are exceptions to this rule. Radiation therapy may be used after a mastectomy if your doctor suspects that the cancer has metastasized to the pectoral muscles or nearby tissue outside the breast. Recent data also suggest that radiation therapy after mastectomy may improve prognosis for women who have node-positive cancers.

How long does radiation therapy usually last?

If you undergo radiation therapy, you will probably have one session a day (5 days a week) for about 6 weeks. Each session lasts only a few minutes. Before radiation therapy begins, you will go in for an initial visit during which your doctor will determine where to target the radiation. X-rays, mammography (a procedure that uses low-dose radiation to create images of the inside of the breast), or other imaging procedures will be used to map the internal structure of the chest area, including the position of internal organs. These procedures are noninvasive and will not cause any pain. Based on these measurements, calculations are made that will determine where to properly aim the radiation, which is produced and directed by a machine called a linear accelerator. During this initial visit, your doctor will place tiny tattoos on portions of the breast or nearby areas that are to be targeted for radiation. These tattoos look like tiny specks. Your doctor will place the tattoos on the breast that was operated on. Applying the tattoos takes about 15 minutes and may cause a stinging sensation but no significant pain.

If I have radiation therapy, am I going to experience nausea and hair loss?

No. Fatigue is the most common complaint associated with radiation therapy. It affects women to different degrees but does not usually interfere with work or normal activities. You may also notice changes in your skin after a few weeks of radiation therapy. The skin of the breast may redden and there may be swelling in the area due to water retention. Skin that is irradiated may appear thicker and the texture of the nipple may feel different than usual. The swelling and skin changes usually go away in 6 months to 1 year. Radiation can slightly increase the risk of lymphedema if you have had an axillary dissection, so you must be even more careful about injury or infections occurring in the hand or arm. In very rare cases, radiation therapy may cause sarcoma (cancer of the connective tissue).

What is breast cancer staging?

Once you have had initial surgery for breast cancer, in the form of breast-conserving surgery or a mastectomy, your breast cancer can be staged according to the classification system known as TNM, where T = tumor size, N = lymph node involvement, and M = metastasis to other parts of the body such as the lungs or bones. Designed by the American Joint Committee on Cancer (AJCC), the TNM system is an objective set of criteria used by doctors to measure the extent of your breast cancer and help you and your doctor decide what further treatments may be necessary, such as systemic therapy in the form of chemotherapy or a hormonal therapy such as tamoxifen (Nolvadex).

- **Stage 0.** This stage includes:
  - DCIS
  - Lobular carcinoma in situ (LCIS)
  - Paget's disease (a cancer affecting the nipple and areola that is usually associated with an underlying carcinoma) without the presence of a tumor

  Treatment for an in situ cancer depends on whether you have DCIS or LCIS. Because DCIS may lead to an invasive ductal carcinoma in the future, many women choose to have breast-conserving surgery to remove the cancer. If the tumor is large or you have cancerous lesions or microcalcifications located in different portions of the breast, a simple mastectomy may be necessary. No immediate treatment is usually recommended for women with LCIS, which is not viewed as a true cancer but rather as a marker lesion that increases the risk of developing an invasive cancer (ductal or lobular) in either breast at some point in the future. If you have LCIS you and your doctor must carefully monitor the health of your breasts—this means annual mammography and a clinical breast exam about three times a year in addition to monthly breast self-exams (BSEs). Some women with LCIS who have other risk factors for breast cancer choose to have a bilateral simple mastectomy,

Breast Cancer Survival by Stage	
Stage	**Percentage of women alive after 5 years from time of diagnosis**
0	100
I	98
2A	88
2B	76
3A	56
3B	49
4	16

Source: Adapted from American Cancer Society, Inc.

which involves the removal of both breasts.

- **Stage 1.** This stage includes:
  - A cancer that is 2 cm ($^3/_4$ in.) or less at its widest point and appears to be confined within the breast

Stage 1 cancer can be treated with either breast-conserving surgery followed by radiation therapy or a modified radical mastectomy. If the tumor is larger than 1 cm (about $^1/_2$ in.) or has unfavorable cellular features such as a high grade or S-phase fraction (a number assigned to a tumor that indicates its growth rate), systemic therapy may be recommended.

- **Stage 2.** This stage includes:
  - A cancer that is 2 cm ($^3/_4$ in.) or less at its widest point and has metastasized to the axillary lymph nodes
  - A cancer that is between 2 and 5 cm (over 2 in.) and may or may not have metastasized to the axillary lymph nodes
  - A cancer that is larger than 5 cm and has not metastasized to the axillary lymph nodes

A Detailed Look at Breast Cancer Staging

Stage Groupings

Stage	Tumor	Node	Metastasis
Stage 0	Tis	N0	M0
Stage I	T1	N0	M0
Stage 2A	T0	N1	M0
	T1	N1	M0
	T2	N0	M0
Stage 2B	T2	N1	M0
	T3	N0	M0
Stage 3A	T0	N2	M0
	T1	N2	M0
	T2	N2	M0
	T3	N2	M0
	T3	N1	M0
	T3	N2	M0
Stage 3B	T4	Any N	M0
	Any T	N3	M0
Stage 4	Any T	Any N	M1

TNM Categories

Primary tumor (T)

TX   Primary tumor cannot be assessed

T0   No evidence of primary tumor

Tis Carcinoma in situ; intraductal carcinoma, LCIS, or Paget's disease of the nipple with no associated tumor mass

T1   Tumor 2.0 cm or less in greatest dimension

T2   Tumor more than 2.0 cm but not more than 5.0 cm in greatest dimension

T3   Tumor more than 5.0 cm in greatest dimension

T4   Tumor of any size with direct extension to chest wall or skin

Regional lymph node involvement (N)

NX Regional lymph nodes cannot be assessed (if they were previously removed, for example)

N0 No regional lymph node metastasis

N1 Metastasis to movable ipsilateral (same side as the breast cancer) axillary lymph node(s)

N2 Metastasis to ipsilateral lymph node(s) fixed to one another or to other structures

N3 Metastasis to ipsilateral internal mammary lymph node(s)

Distant metastasis (M)

MX Presence of distant metastasis cannot be assessed

M0 No distant metastasis

M1 Distant metastasis present, includes metastasis to ipsilateral supraclavicular (above the collarbone) lymph nodes

Source: Adapted from AJCC Cancer Staging Manual, 5th ed., 1997, published by Lippincott-Raven, Philadelphia.

Like a stage 1 cancer, a stage 2 cancer can be treated with either breast-conserving surgery followed by radiation therapy or a modified radical mastectomy. Radiation may be recommended following a modified radical mastectomy depending on the size of the tumor and how many lymph nodes are affected (if any). Systemic therapy is usually recommended following initial surgery for a stage 2 cancer. High-dose chemotherapy may be considered if a large number of lymph nodes are affected.

- **Stage 3.** This stage includes:
    - A cancer that is smaller than 5 cm (5 cm is about

2 in.) at its widest point, has metastasized to the
axillary lymph nodes, and these lymph nodes are
attached to each other or to other structures under the arm
- A cancer that is larger than 5 cm and has metastasized to the axillary lymph nodes
- A cancer that has metastasized to the pectoral
muscles, ribs, or to lymph nodes located near the
sternum (breast bone)

Breast-conserving surgery, a modified radical mastectomy, or a radical mastectomy may be recommended as initial surgery for a tumor classified
as stage 3, followed by radiation therapy (in many
cases) and systemic therapy. High-dose chemotherapy may be considered in the case of a stage 3
cancer that has metastasized to the pectoral muscles, ribs, or to lymph nodes located near the sternum. Systemic therapy may be used before
surgery to shrink a large stage 3 tumor.

- **Stage 4.** This stage includes:
  - A cancer that has metastasized to distant parts of
  the body such as the lungs or bones
  - A cancer that has metastasized to lymph nodes
  located near the collarbone

The main treatment for a stage 4 cancer is systemic
therapy. Surgery or radiation therapy may be used
to help alleviate symptoms. High-dose chemotherapy is also an option.

FIVE

WHAT IS TAMOXIFEN?

QUICK FACT

Tamoxifen has been used for over 20 years to treat breast cancer and in 1998 was shown to reduce the risk of developing the disease.

Rachel, age 68, is a retiree whose experience with breast cancer and tamoxifen began several years ago as she was getting dressed one morning. While buttoning her blouse, she discovered a lump in her right breast that felt hard. Rachel ignored the problem for a few weeks before informing her doctor, who referred her to me. During her visit Rachel admitted that until now she had not been very concerned about the health of her breasts. She had not had a mammogram (an x-ray of the breast) for a number of years and was not in the habit of doing breast self-exams (BSEs). I took Rachel's medical history, examined the lump by palpation (feel), and ordered a mammogram. Based on these initial findings, I was fairly certain that Rachel's tumor (a mass of abnormal cells that may be either cancerous or benign) was cancerous. The next step was a needle biopsy (the removal and analysis of a tissue sample) which, due to the size of the tumor and its location near the surface of the breast, was performed without the aid of mammography (a procedure that uses low-dose radiation to create images of the inside of the breast) or sonography (the use of high-frequency sound waves to create an image of the inside of the body). The biopsy revealed the presence of an invasive

83

ductal carcinoma—a cancerous tumor originating in a milk duct that has broken through the confines of the duct and invaded surrounding breast tissue. An invasive cancer has the potential to metastasize (spread) to nearby axillary (underarm) lymph nodes and to more distant parts of the body such as the lungs or bones. Rachel's tumor appeared to be about 2 cm wide (the size of a nickel) and was located in the upper, outer quadrant of her breast. Chances are that a screening mammogram would have brought this abnormality to her attention years before it became palpable. Fortunately for Rachel, breast cancers that strike women her age tend to grow more slowly than those in younger women. We were able to start treating her disease before it had progressed to the point of being life-threatening.

Rachel underwent a quadranectomy (a breast conserving surgical procedure similar to a lumpectomy except that it removes more tissue—about 25% of the breast). The accompanying axillary dissection (a surgical procedure that involves the removal of axillary lymph nodes adjacent to the affected breast in order to determine if a breast cancer has metastasized to the lymph nodes and how many are affected) revealed that her cancer was node-negative—the cancer had not spread to the lymph nodes. Because of the location of her tumor, which was fairly close to the axilla (armpit), the surgeon was able to remove the lymph nodes without making an additional incision. I explained to Rachel that radiation therapy was required to complete local treatment and eradicate whatever was left of the cancer in her breast. We also discussed the prospect of adjuvant therapy (additional therapy after primary treatment) with tamoxifen. Rachel's cancer was grade 2 (grade is a number from 1 to 3, rating the ability of cancer cells to divide and grow, that helps to distinguish slower-growing from more aggressive tumors) and characterized by the presence of aneuploid cells (cells that contain an abnormal amount of material in their nuclei). While the node-negative status of Rachel's cancer significantly improved her prognosis (outlook for recovery), the size of her tumor and its cellular features indicated the need for systemic (whole body) treatment to prevent a recurrence or metastasis. Tests of hormone receptor status indicated that Rachel would probably benefit from tamoxifen therapy. Her tumor was not only estrogen receptor positive but also contained high levels of estrogen receptor proteins. I explained to Rachel that tamoxifen has been shown to reduce the risk of recurrence by 60% in women her age with such high levels of estrogen receptors. She expressed some concern over the serious side effects associated with tamoxifen and wanted to know if these risks applied equally to everyone. I explained that as a nonsmoker in good general health—Rachel had no history of hypertension (high blood pressure) or blood clots— she was not at great risk for developing vascular (blood vessel) problems such as pulmonary embolism (a blood clot in the arteries to the lungs). Because Rachel had undergone a hysterectomy (the surgical removal of the uterus) years ago, endometrial cancer (cancer of the lining of the uterus) was not a consideration. Rachel took a few weeks to make her decision. Ultimately she opted to start on tamoxifen therapy as the best way to remain disease free.

The rise of tamoxifen (Nolvadex) from a failed birth control pill to the most frequently prescribed anticancer medication in the world began over 30 years ago in a pharmaceutical company laboratory. The results of animal studies convinced researchers that tamoxifen would not work as a contraceptive, but soon afterward they discovered that the medication has antiestrogenic (estrogen-blocking) properties in breast tissue. This was a crucial step in the development of tamoxifen as a breast cancer treatment. Doctors knew that estrogen, the primary female sex hormone, can fuel the growth of certain cancerous tumors in the breast and quickly recognized the potential of an estrogen-stopper such as tamoxifen. Between the late 1970s and today, tamoxifen has been the subject of a series of Food and Drug Administration (FDA) approvals and has become the most popular hormonal therapy used in the fight against breast cancer—from small tumors to advanced forms of the disease. Taken in pill form, tamoxifen is often used after initial surgery for early breast cancer (cancers that are confined to the breast or that have spread only as far as the underarm lymph nodes), especially in women who have cancers that are estrogen receptor positive (cancers whose growth is stimulated by estrogen). Women with estrogen receptor positive tumors who take tamoxifen for several years after breast cancer surgery are much less likely to experience a recurrence or to die from the disease. Doctors also rely upon tamoxifen to help control metastatic disease—breast cancer that has traveled through the bloodstream or lymphatic system (the system of organs and tissues that are vital to your body's ability to fight infection and disease) to take root in distant parts of the body such as vital organs or bones.

Despite the fact that tamoxifen has been studied for decades as a breast cancer treatment, doctors are still unlocking the potential of this powerful medication. This became clear in late 1998 when tamoxifen was shown to be the first medication in history that may be able to stop breast cancer before it starts. Tamoxifen's long-studied effectiveness in treating all stages of breast cancer—and the fact that in previous studies tamoxifen appeared to reduce the risk of developing a *new* cancer in the opposite breast— had led many experts to suspect that tamoxifen might be able to prevent the disease in women at high risk. In the early 1990s, researchers put this theory to the test by study-ing the use of tamoxifen in thousands of healthy women who were at high risk for breast cancer due to age, family history of breast cancer, or other factors. After about 5 years of study, the findings suggest that women at high risk for breast cancer who take tamoxifen are nearly 50% less likely to develop the disease. These findings offer new hope for women who are concerned about their risk for breast cancer. Until now, these women were forced to take a wait-and-see approach toward the possibility of breast cancer development—an approach that includes close monitoring of the breasts through regular mammography (a procedure that uses low-dose radiation to create images of the inside of the breast) and clinical breast exams—or to undergo prophylactic mastectomy (the removal of one or both breasts before evidence of cancer is present in order to prevent the onset of the disease).

Doctors know more today about what tamoxifen can do than ever before. They also know more about how the medication works and the effects that it has on a woman's body as a whole. These days doctors believe that tamoxifen not only has antiestrogenic properties but estrogenic (estrogenlike) powers as well. Simply put, tamoxifen has the ability to act like estrogen in some parts of the body while blocking its effects in others—what doctors refer to as a selective estrogen receptor modulator (SERM). Tamoxifen inhibits estrogen in breast cancer cells that have receptors for the hormone—these receptors are the "docking ports" through which estrogen binds to and communicates with the cells—and mimics estrogen in other parts of the body such as bones and blood vessels. Unlike the surgery or radiation therapy often used as initial treatment for breast cancer—each of which is a local therapy designed to eradicate cancerous cells from the breast or chest region—tamoxifen is a systemic (whole body) therapy. It cannot be "aimed at" or focused on breast tissue or limited to specific regions of the body. Once in your bloodstream, tamoxifen roams freely throughout your circulatory system. In bone and blood vessels, tamoxifen has a healthy, estrogenlike effect. The result is usually stronger bones and a healthier heart. Unfortunately, tamoxifen acts like an estrogen in the uterus as well, where it may stimulate a benign (noncancerous) overgrowth of tissue or even the development of cancer. See

Chapter 8 for more information on tamoxifen's effects on bone and heart health.

What is tamoxifen primarily used for today?

Tamoxifen has been used for decades to treat various stages of breast cancer and is now poised to become an important first line of defense for women who are at high risk for the disease. For many women, the question of whether to use tamoxifen arises after initial surgery for breast cancer. As you saw in Chapter 4, the initial treatment for most breast cancers involves some form of surgery to remove the cancer from the breast and sample axillary (underarm) lymph nodes for the presence of cancerous cells. About 1 month to 6 weeks after surgery many women receive adjuvant therapy (additional therapy used after primary treatment). The purpose of adjuvant therapy for breast cancer—which usually involves systemic therapy in the form of hormonal therapy or chemotherapy—is to eliminate any cancerous cells that remain in the breast or that have begun to metastasize (spread) to other parts of the body. After surgery and radiation therapy are used to treat a breast cancer, there may be very tiny amounts of cancerous cells in your breast or in other parts of your body that cannot be detected—even with the sensitive, high-tech equipment used today. If your doctor waits until these cancerous cells become detectable, it may be too late to address the problem effectively.

Adjuvant therapy is a preemptive strike designed mainly to combat the possible recurrence of breast cancer or keep it from metastasizing. Whether your doctor recommends adjuvant therapy for you after surgery depends on the nature of your breast cancer profile, which is developed after a tumor is removed and also during the initial needle or excisional biopsy. The main factors in this decision, or profile, include the size of your tumor and other prognostic indicators such as the cellular features discussed in Chapter 3. Doctors generally consider the use of adjuvant therapy based on the risk of recurrence or metastasis. If this risk is estimated to be greater than 10 to 15%, adjuvant therapy is often prescribed. Women with a risk of recurrence or metastasis that is less than 10 to 15% can usually be spared adjuvant therapy because the potential benefits do not outweigh the risks posed by side effects. If you have a breast cancer with estrogen receptors, your doctor may prescribe tamoxifen after breast cancer surgery if your cancer has metastasized to the lymph nodes or is greater than 1 cm and has unfavorable cellular features such as high grade (a number from one to three, rating the ability of cancer cells to divide and grow, that helps to distinguish slower-growing from more aggressive tumors).

Is tamoxifen effective as adjuvant therapy?

Yes. Years of medical studies suggest that in women of all ages tamoxifen is very effective at preventing recurrence and reducing a woman's risk of ultimately dying from breast cancer due to a metastasis. Tamoxifen can also help to prevent a contralateral breast cancer (the development of a new breast cancer in the opposite breast). Curbing the risk of a contralateral breast cancer is an important potential benefit of tamoxifen, because having breast cancer increases your risk of developing a contralateral breast cancer by three or four times. In women with breast cancers that are estrogen receptor positive, 5 years of adjuvant therapy with tamoxifen can reduce:

- Risk of recurrence by about 50%

- Risk of dying from breast cancer by 28%

- Risk of developing a contralateral breast cancer by approximately 47%

As you can see, tamoxifen offers significant protection in a number of important areas—protection that does not fade once treatment ends. Studies suggest that these benefits last for at least 5 to 10 years after use of tamoxifen is stopped. Because tamoxifen works primarily by blocking the cancer-fueling effects of estrogen, it is much more effective in women who have cancers that are estrogen receptor positive. (As you saw in Chapter 1, postmenopausal women are more likely than younger women to have breast cancers that contain estrogen receptors.) In women whose breast cancers do not have these receptors, tamoxifen has been shown to lower rates of recurrence by 10% and mortality rates by 6%. Tamoxifen can be used alone or combined with chemotherapy. In women who have completed menopause, this combination is more effective in preventing breast cancer recurrence than tamoxifen or chemotherapy alone (this is not the case in women under age 50). While some studies suggest that the combination of tamoxifen and chemotherapy can reduce the risk of recurrence 28% more than using tamoxifen alone, this powerful duo does not appear to produce survival rates higher than those achieved by using single-agent tamoxifen therapy. See Chapter 6 for information on using tamoxifen as adjuvant therapy.

Can tamoxifen be used to treat breast cancers that have metastasized to distant parts of the body?

Yes. In fact, tamoxifen has been used for over 20 years to treat metastatic breast cancer. In women with stage 4 breast cancers that are estrogen receptor positive, tamoxifen is often an important part of an overall therapeutic strategy. This strategy—which may also include chemotherapy, other hormonal therapies, radiation therapy, and limited surgery—is aimed at alleviating symptoms, preventing complications, and maintaining the highest quality of life possible with respect to the severity of the disease. Tamoxifen is often considered a first choice of treatment in women of every age who have metastatic cancer and are good candidates for hormonal therapy. Why? Because about 60 to 75% of women with cancers that are estrogen receptor positive respond to therapy with tamoxifen. Women with estrogen receptor negative breast cancers respond less

well to tamoxifen—it benefits perhaps 10 to 20% of these
women. Eventually most women who are helped by tamoxifen develop a resistance to its therapeutic effects. When
this happens, other hormonal therapies or chemotherapy
may be tried. Women who have a response to tamoxifen
often benefit from another hormonal medication once
tamoxifen resistance has developed—sometimes three or
four hormonal therapies are used in sequence to check the
progress of the disease. By using all available treatments, it
is possible to manage metastatic cancer anywhere from

**The Evolution of Tamoxifen: Important
FDA Approvals**

- **Metastatic breast cancer.** In the late
1970s, tamoxifen was introduced in the United States as a treatment for metastatic breast
cancer in postmenopausal women. The medication was approved for premenopausal
women with this form of the disease about
10 years later.

- **Adjuvant therapy.** In the mid-1980s,
tamoxifen was approved for use as adjuvant therapy in postmenopausal women with
node-positive breast cancers (cancers that
have metastasized at least as far as the axillary lymph nodes), alone or in conjunction
with chemotherapy. Tamoxifen was approved
in 1990 as adjuvant therapy for node-negative
breast cancers (cancers that are confined to
the breast and do not involve metastasis to
the axillary lymph nodes) regardless of menopausal status.

- **Risk reduction.** In 1998 tamoxifen was approved for use in women at high risk of
developing breast cancer.

months to years. Ultimately most women with metastic cancer fall victim to the disease. See Chapter 6 for more information on metastatic cancer and the use of tamoxifen to treat it.

My doctor says that tamoxifen has not been proven to prevent breast cancer, only to reduce the risk. What's the difference?

That is an excellent question. The distinction between prevention and risk reduction is an important one and may be easy for some women to overlook in the flurry of excitement surrounding the new use of this decades-old medication. At issue here is the question of whether tamoxifen is truly a chemopreventive agent (a medication or other substance that has the power to prevent cancer development). Unfortunately the answer is still an unknown. The fact is that we know a lot more about tamoxifen as a treatment for breast cancer than we do about its possible preventive powers. Let us briefly survey what we know. Tamoxifen is approved by the FDA for reducing the risk of breast cancer in women who are likely to develop the disease. The decision of the FDA was based largely on the results of a medical study called the National Surgical Adjuvant Breast and Bowel Project (NSABP) Breast Cancer Prevention Trial, which was sponsored by the National Cancer Institute (NCI). In this study, over 13,000 women age 35 or over at high risk for breast cancer took tamoxifen or a placebo (sugar pill) for 5 years. The degree of risk was calculated in several ways. Women age 60 or over were allowed to participate in the trial based on age alone. Women under age 60 were eligible if they had high-risk profiles based on some of the factors described in Chapter 2. The trial was stopped 14 months early in order to give women in the placebo group a chance to switch to tamoxifen.

The study results, published in the *Journal of the National Cancer Institute* in 1998, suggest that tamoxifen reduced the risk of developing breast cancer in these women by a significant 49%. What does this study actually tell us? It indicates that tamoxifen reduced the risk of cancer development during the 5 years that the study was conducted. It does not tell us anything about the long-term protection provided by tamoxifen—and this is what we need to know in order to say with certainty that tamoxifen actually prevents breast cancer. We do not know at this point whether taking tamoxifen for several years only delays the appearance of cancer because long-term studies have not yet been con-

---

Tamoxifen and Breast Cancer

- **Adjuvant therapy.** In women whose breast cancers contain estrogen receptors, 5 years of tamoxifen therapy after initial surgery can reduce the risk of recurrence by about 50% and the risk of dying from breast cancer by 28%. Women who take the medication are also 47% less likely to develop a contralateral breast cancer. Tamoxifen is effective regardless of axillary lymph node status and has its greatest effect in women whose cancers are sensitive to the effects of estrogen.

- **Metastatic breast cancer.** Tamoxifen is used in women with cancers that have metastasized to distant parts of the body in order to help control the extent and severity of the disease. About 60 to 75% of women whose breast cancers contain estrogen receptors have a positive response to tamoxifen. Even 10 to 20% of women whose cancers do not contain estrogen receptors have a favorable response to the medication.

- **Risk reduction.** In women who do not have breast cancer but are likely to develop it, tamoxifen can reduce breast cancer risk by about 50%.

ducted. Until doctors can follow the progress of the women in this and other studies for 10 or 15 years, most doctors will be hesitant to claim that tamoxifen can prevent breast cancer. See Chapter 7 for information on taking tamoxifen to reduce your risk of developing breast cancer.

How does tamoxifen work against breast cancer?

Tamoxifen is effective in treating breast cancer and reducing the risk for the disease because of its antiestrogenic properties. While estrogen, which is a naturally-occurring hormone in the female body, has a variety of beneficial effects and is vital to good health, it also has the unfortunate power to fuel the growth of certain breast cancers. It accomplishes this by binding to the estrogen receptors on the surface of cancerous cells. As you saw in Chapter 1, hormones such as estrogen are chemical message carriers that fit into cell receptors (the way keys fit into locks) and stimulate or suppress activity within cells. How does estrogen encourage the growth of breast cancer? No one knows for certain, but the answer may involve growth factors. Growth factors are proteins that help to regulate cell growth. In breast cancer cells that are estrogen receptor positive, estrogen appears to influence the actions of certain growth factors that control cell proliferation (growth). These include transforming growth factor (TGF) alpha, TGF beta, and insulin-like growth factor (IGF). TGF alpha and IGF accelerate cell growth, while TGF beta acts as a brake on runaway cell proliferation. When estrogen chemically interfaces with cancerous cells via the receptors on their surfaces, it appears to stimulate the production of TGF alpha and IGF while suppressing levels of TGF beta. By accelerating cell growth and releasing the molecular brakes, estrogen encourages the proliferation of cancerous cells. The result is a larger tumor or a dangerous metastasis. This is where tamoxifen enters the picture. Tamoxifen blocks estrogen by binding to the estrogen receptors, preventing the hormone from chemically connecting to cancerous cells. About 65 to 80% of breast cancers in postmenopausal women contain receptors for estrogen. Those statistics fall to 45 to 60% for premenopausal women.

If tamoxifen works by blocking estrogen, why does it have any effect at all on breast cancers without estrogen receptors?

That is a good question. Your instincts are correct—tamoxifen does appear to do more than just block estrogen from binding to receptors. Tamoxifen is most effective when used in women who have cancers that are estrogen receptor positive. The benefit for women with estrogen receptor negative breast cancers is minimal. But the fact that tamoxifen produces even a small benefit in the latter group of women has led doctors to speculate that the medication has other mechanisms of action as well (mechanisms of action are the processes by which a medication produces its effects). Why does tamoxifen appear to provide a small amount of protection to women without estrogen receptors on their breast cancer cells? When tamoxifen binds with estrogen receptors on the surface of a cancerous cell, it literally occupies the receptor "docking ports" so that estrogen cannot chemically communicate with the cell. But tamoxifen may do more than just provide good defense. It may be sending messages of its own to the inside of the cell—messages very different from those carried by estrogen. Whereas estrogen stimulates the production of TGF alpha and IGF—the growth factors that promote cell proliferation—tamoxifen may signal a slowdown of these growth factors. Tamoxifen may also step up production of TGF beta, which is the molecular brake on the out-of-control cell growth characteristic of cancer. Tamoxifen may combat cancer in other ways as well. It may increase the production of what doctors refer to as natural killer cells—a specialized, elite core of white blood cells marshaled by the immune system to attack tumors or viruses. Tamoxifen may increase blood levels of globulin (a type of protein), which tends to bind to estrogen and thus may reduce the amount of circulating hormone available to feed the growth of can-

How Tamoxifen Affects Different Parts of the Body

Your doctor may prescribe tamoxifen to prevent breast cancer from recurring or metastasizing or to reduce the risk of developing the disease, but it is also important to understand how this systemic medication affects your body as a whole.

- **Breast.** In the breast, tamoxifen acts like an estrogen blocker. It can help to prevent a breast cancer from recurring or metastasizing and can reduce the likelihood of the disease in healthy women at high risk.

- **Bones.** Tamoxifen acts like estrogen in bone, where estrogen has a healthy, bone-building effect. Tamoxifen can help to preserve or increase bone density in postmenopausal women for as long as they take the medication. In women who have not completed menopause, tamoxifen may actually speed bone loss.

- **Heart.** By mimicking estrogen in blood vessels, tamoxifen has been shown to reduce total cholesterol and low density lipoprotein (LDL) levels. Tamoxifen's healthy effects on the heart may provide protection against heart disease for as long as you take the medication.

- **Uterus.** Unfortunately, tamoxifen appears to act like an estrogen in the uterus. There, tamoxifen can stimulate an overgrowth of tissue in the uterus and may increase the risk of endometrial cancer (cancer of the lining of the uterus).

cerous cells. Finally, tamoxifen may inhibit an enzyme called protein kinase C that is associated with cell growth.

Is tamoxifen just another kind of estrogen therapy?

No. Although tamoxifen is a hormonal medication, it and other SERMs are different from the estrogen therapy used by women after menopause. Tamoxifen is different from estrogen replacement therapy (ERT) and hormone replacement therapy (HRT)—a combination of estrogen and progesterone—both in terms of chemistry and the effect on the body. Tamoxifen acts like estrogen in some parts of the body while blocking its effects in others. Estrogen therapy, on the other hand, is a way of restoring the estrogen lost due to menopause, and estrogen therapy does not have the ability to "decide" when to act like estrogen and when not to.

ERT and HRT are used to ease the symptoms of menopause and to prevent or treat serious conditions that women are often more susceptible to as they grow older. Estrogen therapy can ease hot flashes (sudden rushes of warmth, lasting anywhere from several seconds to several minutes and varying in intensity, that start in the chest and radiate into the neck and face), night sweats (hot flashes that occur at night during sleep), and vaginal dryness. It maintains strong bones and reduces the risk of heart disease. Recent research also indicates that ERT and HRT may reduce the incidence of Alzheimer's disease and improve mood and memory changes often seen at menopause.

Does tamoxifen have any serious side effects?

Yes. While the most common side effects of tamoxifen— such as hot flashes and vaginal bleeding—can be classified as little more than bothersome, this medication is also associated with a number of rare but serious side effects including endometrial cancer (cancer of the lining of the uterus). The NCI, like most national health organizations, does

Common Side Effects of Tamoxifen

The short-term side effects associated with tamoxifen are generally mild and better tolerated than those reported by women on chemotherapy. Only about 5% of women who take tamoxifen to treat breast cancer stop taking it due to its side effects. Hot flashes are the most common complaint. Other side effects include:

- Vaginal discharge or bleeding
- Irregular menstrual periods
- Irritation of the skin around the vagina
- Weight gain
- Headache
- Dizziness
- Fatigue
- Loss of appetite

emphasize that the benefits of using tamoxifen as a breast cancer treatment outweigh the risks associated with the medication.

- **Endometrial cancer.** By acting like estrogen in the uterus, tamoxifen has a stimulating effect on the tissue there. This can lead to the development of hyperplasia (an excessive growth of abnormal cells) or polyps (growths originating in mucous membranes that are usually benign but can be cancerous). In more serious cases the stimulating effect of tamoxifen on the uterus can lead to endometrial cancer. Medical studies suggest that taking tamoxifen for about 5 years can increase your risk for this type of cancer by two to three times. Age appears to be a contributing factor as well. Most women who develop endometrial cancer while taking tamoxifen are age 50 or over. Most cases of endometrial cancer that occur in women taking tamoxifen are detected at early stages when they can be treated most effectively, though some have been fatal. If you are taking tamoxifen, you should have annual gynecologic exams and always report irregular periods, vaginal bleeding or discharge, or pelvic pain or pressure to your doctor.

- **Blood clots.** Taking tamoxifen may increase by several times your risk of developing pulmonary embolism or deep vein thrombosis—both of which can cause serious health problems and even death. Women who have had blood clots in the past are more likely to experience them while taking tamoxifen, as are women age 50 or over. Combining tamoxifen with chemotherapy may also increase the risk of a blood clot. If you have had blood clots in the past or suspect that you may be spending long periods of time confined to bed while on tamoxifen, you should discuss the risk of blood clots with your doctor before using the medication.

  - A pulmonary embolism is a blood clot in the arteries to the lungs. The clot usually originates in a vein in the leg or pelvis and travels to the lungs via the bloodstream. Once in the lungs, a large clot can cause death in minutes by cutting off blood circulation in the organ. A small clot is not immediately fatal but can cause damage to the lung. Symptoms of a pulmonary embolism including breathing difficulties, chest pain, and coughing up of blood.

  - Deep vein thrombosis refers to a blood clot in

the deep veins of the legs or pelvis. Being confined to bed or experiencing a leg injury can increase your risk of this kind of clot. Deep vein thrombosis often causes pain or swelling in the area of the clot.

- **Stroke.** Tamoxifen slightly increases the risk of stroke. A stroke occurs due to an interruption of the blood supply to the brain or part of the brain, resulting in brain damage. The interruption is usually caused by a blockage in an artery or the rupturing of a blood vessel.

- **Eye problems.** Taking tamoxifen may slightly increase your risk of developing cataracts (a clouding of the lens of the eye) or worsen existing cataracts. Women who have had cataracts in the past are more at risk. Tamoxifen is also associated with retinopathy (disorders of the retina) and changes in color perception. If you are taking tamoxifen, you should have your eyes examined by an ophthalmologist (a doctor who treats diseases of the eye) every 2 years. Changes in vision should always be reported to your doctor.

- **Liver problems.** In a small number of women, using tamoxifen may lead to the development of liver problems such as cholestasis (the failure of the liver to produce amounts of bile sufficient for proper digestion), hepatitis (liver inflammation), and hepatic necrosis (the death of liver tissue). In a Swedish study in which women took 40 mg of tamoxifen daily for 2 to 5 years, three cases of liver cancer were reported in the tamoxifen group (one case occurred in the placebo group). Tamoxifen has not been linked to liver cancer in other human studies of the medication. If you take tamoxifen, your

---

Rare but Serious Side Effects Associated with Tamoxifen

- Endometrial cancer
- Pulmonary embolism
- Deep vein thrombosis
- Stroke
- Liver problems
- Cataracts
- Retinopathy
- Depression

---

doctor may wish to order blood tests periodically to check your liver function.

- **Depression.** The link between tamoxifen and depression appears to be thin. In one study, depression was reported by 1% of women taking the medication. This side effect has not been reported in other studies.

The number and severity of side effects associated with tamoxifen vary from woman to woman and depend to some extent on your medical history, your age, and whether you are using tamoxifen as adjuvant therapy or for metastatic cancer or risk reduction. Chapters 6 and 7 also take a closer look at medical studies involving tamoxifen and the side effects experienced by the women who participated.

SIX

USING TAMOXIFEN AS ADJUVANT THERAPY OR TO TREAT METASTATIC BREAST CANCER

QUICK FACT

If your breast cancer is estrogen receptor positive, 5 years of adjuvant therapy with tamoxifen may reduce your risk of breast cancer recurrence by 50%.

Though we cannot yet cure metastatic breast cancer, which occurs when cancer cells in the breast invade distant parts of the body such as the lungs or bones, women with the disease are living longer and enjoying a higher quality of life today thanks to effective treatments such as tamoxifen (Nolvadex). Delores, age 42, is a fifth-grade schoolteacher who experienced bone metastases years after her initial treatment for breast cancer. She is the third woman in her family diagnosed with the disease. Delores' mother is a breast cancer survivor and her older sister died of this type of cancer. Despite close monitoring of the breasts, Delores was diagnosed over 7 years ago with invasive lobular carcinoma, a cancer that has spread from its original site in a lobule (milk-producing gland) and invaded surrounding breast tissue and possibly other parts of the body. Three axillary (underarm) lymph nodes were affected. Breast cancers in premenopausal women such as Delores tend to develop faster than those affecting women her mother's age. The breast tissue of younger women is also denser, making it more difficult for radiologists (doctors trained in the interpretation of x-ray and other images) to detect small abnormalities on their mammograms (x-rays of the breast). Local treatment of Dolores' cancer consisted of breast-conserving surgery with axillary dissection—a surgical procedure that involves the removal of the axillary lymph nodes adjacent to the affected breast in order to determine if a breast cancer has metastasized to the lymph nodes and how many are affected—followed by 6 weeks of radiation therapy. Dolores also received six cycles of CMF, a popular chemotherapy regimen for breast cancer.

Disease free for 6 years, Dolores thought that her battle with breast cancer was behind her until she began experiencing bone pain about 10 months ago. Based on her symptoms I suspected that her cancer had returned. A bone scan soon revealed metastases to the bones of the ribs, spine, and hips. A bone scan, which is an imaging procedure that can be used to pinpoint the location of cancerous cells in the skeleton, involves injecting a low-dose radioactive dye into a vein and then taking images. Abnormalities show up as radioactive hotspots. I was concerned that the cancer might have weakened some of the affected bones, leaving them vulnerable to fracture. Some x-rays were taken in order to assess the strength of Dolores' bones, after which I concluded that she was not at risk for an impending fracture. This was an important finding because even slight trauma, such as that resulting from a minor fall or even stepping off a curb, can cause fragile bones to break. I also ordered blood tests and additional imaging procedures to determine if the cancer had infiltrated other parts of Dolores' body. It had not.

Dolores was a good candidate for hormonal therapy—her cancer was estrogen receptor positive—and I recommended starting her on tamoxifen. (Bone metastases after such a long disease-free interval is often a telltale indication that a cancer has estrogen receptors.) Tamoxifen was the right choice for a couple of reasons. Dolores had not taken tamoxifen after her initial breast cancer surgery (if she had, taking tamoxifen during the time that her cancer was spreading might not have produced a favorable response) and tamoxifen is particularly effective when used to combat metastases in bone. Dolores had only been taking tamoxifen for about 5 days when she began to experience bone pain again. She was alarmed and assumed that her disease was getting worse. I explained that the onset of bone pain during the first month or so of hormonal therapy—doctors refer to this phenomenon as a flare—is often an indication that the medication is working. I prescribed a pain reliever to ease these temporary aches, which began to fade after about 6 weeks. Six months later I was pleased to inform Dolores that another bone scan revealed improvement in her condition. Untroubled for now by symptoms or medication side effects, Dolores continues to teach and spends as much time as she can with her husband and two children.

———

As you saw in Chapter 4, the initial treatment for most breast cancers involves some form of surgery—breast-conserving surgery or mastectomy—to remove the cancer from the breast and sample axillary (underarm) lymph nodes for the presence of cancerous cells. Surgery for breast cancer, as well as the radiation therapy that often accompanies breast-conserving procedures, is considered local treatment because its purpose is to eliminate the tumor (a mass of abnormal cells that may be either cancerous or benign) from the breast while leaving the rest of the body unaffected. Many women also receive adjuvant therapy, which is additional therapy used after primary treatment, beginning about 1 month to 6 weeks after their operations.

Adjuvant therapy, in the form of hormonal therapy or chemotherapy, is a systemic (whole body) treatment designed to eliminate any cancerous cells that remain in the breast or that have begun to metastasize (spread) to other parts of the body. These residual cells, inhabiting the breast or more distant regions of the body, may exist in such tiny amounts that they cannot be detected by high-tech imaging procedures such as mammography (a procedure that uses low-dose radiation to create images of the inside of the breast) or other tests used to detect cancer. It can be an unsettling thought—the idea that microscopic colonies of breast cancer cells may remain in your body after surgery, eluding our best efforts to discover them. This is the problem that adjuvant therapy was created to solve. It is the most effective way to treat these unseen, potentially destructive remnants of a breast cancer. Think of adjuvant therapy as a powerful, preemptive strike engineered to prevent a cancer from coming back or from metastasizing.

But if these residual cancer cells are undetectable, how do women and their doctors know when to use adjuvant therapy? This decision is based on the details of your recurrence risk profile, which is usually complete after your operation. The pathologist's report will reveal the particular character of your breast cancer. What is the size of your tumor? What sort of telltale cellular traits does your breast cancer have? How far has it spread? By answering questions such as these, you and your doctor can assess the possibility that your cancer may return or metastasize. If this risk is estimated to be greater than 10 to 15%, adjuvant therapy is usually in order. (About 70% of women with breast cancer are spared adjuvant therapy after surgery because their risks of recurrence or metastasis are so low that the potential benefits of further treatment are equaled or outweighed by the risks.) If you are diagnosed with a breast cancer that has receptors for estrogen, your doctor may prescribe tamoxifen (Nolvadex) with or without chemotherapy after breast cancer surgery if your tumor has metastasized to the lymph nodes or is greater than 1 cm and has unfavorable cellular features such as high grade—a number from 1 to 3, rating the ability of cancer cells to divide and grow, that helps to distinguish slower-growing from more aggressive tumors.

For over 20 years tamoxifen has also been a source of hope for women whose breast cancers are incurable. These incurable cancers occur when cancerous cells in the breast travel through the bloodstream or lymphatic system, the system of organs and tissues that are vital to your body's ability to fight infection and disease, and take root in distant parts of the body such as vital organs or bones. By helping to control severe forms of breast cancer and easing uncomfortable symptoms, tamoxifen gives many women with metastatic disease the freedom to focus on their lives and not their illnesses. In addition to tamoxifen, an overall treatment program may employ chemotherapy, radiation therapy, and limited surgery to ensure that women with fatal metastases liver longer, better lives. A small number of women effectively manage their disease for a decade or longer.

What is chemotherapy and how is it different from a hormonal therapy such as tamoxifen?

Chemotherapy, which is very effective when used as adjuvant therapy or to treat metastatic breast cancer, involves the use of combinations of powerful anticancer medications that are given intravenously or occasionally by mouth. Chemotherapy medications attack and destroy cancerous cells by damaging their DNA or interfering with cell division during vulnerable stages of cell reproduction. Hormonal therapies like tamoxifen combat estrogen-sensitive breast cancers by starving them of the hormonal fuel they need to grow. Chemotherapy medications are associated with more severe short-term side effects than tamoxifen or most other hormonal therapies. The anticancer medications of chemotherapy—each of which has the power to attack a cancer cell in a different way and at a different point in the cell's reproductive cycle—are most effective when used in combination. Combinations are developed carefully so as to avoid overlapping side effects. The most common chemotherapy regimens used in the treatment of breast cancer are cyclophosphamide (Cytoxan), methotrexate (Rheumatrex), and fluorouracil (5-FU)—this combination is often referred to by the abbreviation CMF—and cyclophosphamide and doxorubicin (Adriamycin) with or without fluorouracil—this combination is often referred to as AC or CAF. Recent studies also suggest that paclitaxel (Taxol), made from the bark of the yew tree, may become an important addition to certain breast cancer chemotherapy regimens used to treat metastatic disease and perhaps early breast cancers (cancers that are confined to the breast or that have spread only as far as the axillary lymph nodes).

While a medication such as tamoxifen is taken daily for a period of years, chemotherapy medications are usually administered in cycles—each lasting about 1 month—with 2 to 4 weeks of chemotherapy-free recovery time between cycles. A typical chemotherapy regimen lasts anywhere

---

Side Effects Associated with Chemotherapy

Side effects vary depending on the drugs that are used.

- Nausea
- Vomiting
- Hair loss
- Loss of appetite
- Mouth sores
- Menstrual irregularities
- Infection (possibly life-threatening)
- Fatigue
- Nerve damage
- Heart muscle damage
- Premature menopause
- Infertility
- Acute myeloid leukemia (AML)

from 3 to 6 months, although in the case of metastatic breast cancer the duration of chemotherapy may vary.

How serious are the side effects associated with chemotherapy?

They range from the merely bothersome to the very serious. The reason that the cancer-killing medications of chemotherapy are often so toxic is that they do not always distinguish between cancerous and healthy cells during their systemic, seek-and-destroy missions. These medications are designed to zero in on the almost hyperactive, out-of-control cell growth associated with cancer. The relatively slow turnover rate of most healthy cells in the body is what protects them from being targeted for destruction by chemotherapy medications. The problem arises because there are other healthy cells in the body that also tend to proliferate at a high rate. The anticancer medications are not sophisticated enough to distinguish between friend and foe as they sweep through the body attacking growing cells. Faster growing, healthy cells—found in bone marrow, hair, and in the gastrointestinal tract—are often the casualties of a chemotherapy offensive. The recovery periods between chemotherapy cycles are intended to give these healthy cells, which retain the ability to repair damage done to them, time to regroup and marshal their forces before subsequent rounds of cancer-killing medications are administered.

What sort of side effects does chemotherapy cause?

It is important to understand that chemotherapy does not affect every woman in the same way. The side effects that you may experience while on chemotherapy depend on which medications are included in your regimen, the dosage being used, your general health, and the duration of treatment. Temporary side effects may include nausea, vomiting, hair loss, loss of appetite, and menstrual irregularities. Many of the side effects that chemotherapy is notorious for in the minds of the American public—such as nausea and vomiting—can usually be controlled or eliminated through the use of other medications such antiemetics. Certain medications frequently included in chemotherapy regimens can also have permanent consequences such as nerve and heart muscle damage and cause the onset of menopause in women in their late 30s or early 40s. The older a woman is when she receives chemotherapy, the greater the risk that she will become infertile or menopausal as a result. Very rarely, the use of certain chemotherapy medications can lead to the development of acute myeloid leukemia (AML)—a life-threatening cancer of the white blood cells— years after breast cancer treatment.

The side effects that usually cause the most concern result from the fact that chemotherapy medications can temporarily suppress the production of stem cells in bone marrow. Stem cells are vital to good health because they are the precursors of red and white blood cells and platelets. Red blood cells carry oxygen from the lungs to other tissues in the body. Low levels of these cells can result in anemia and fatigue. White blood cells help to combat infection. A very low white blood cell count may leave you susceptible to potentially fatal infections. Severe shortages of blood-clotting platelets, which are needed in sufficient amounts to repair damaged blood vessels, can lead to bleeding as a result of relatively minor wounds. These deficiencies in blood cells or platelets can be addressed in several ways. Injections of growth factors (proteins that help to regulate cell growth) can be used to boost white blood cell counts. Platelet transfusions can reduce the risk of bleeding. If anemia is a concern, the hormone erythropoietin (Epogen or Procrit) can be used to increase levels of red blood cells.

What are the main benefits of using tamoxifen as adjuvant therapy?

If your breast cancer has receptors for estrogen, using tamoxifen after your surgery can help you stay alive and cancer free—that is probably the most concise way to sum

High-Dose Chemotherapy, Bone Marrow Transplant, and Stem Cell Transplantation

In the controversial practice of high-dose chemotherapy, large quantities of anticancer medications are administered in one brief cycle. Doctors sometimes recommend high-dose chemotherapy to treat carefully selected women with metastatic breast cancer or women in whom the risk of recurrence is very high after breast cancer surgery. In the not-so-distant past, bone marrow transplant was a necessary adjunct to high-dose chemotherapy. It was and is still sometimes used to spare a portion of bone marrow (the site of stem cell production) from the highly toxic effects of this type of chemotherapy in order to return the bone marrow to the body later. A bone marrow transplant is a two-part surgical procedure that initially requires the use of general anesthesia to remove bone marrow from the hip before high-dose chemotherapy begins. The bone marrow is then replaced via an intravenous (IV) line after the chemotherapy regimen is complete. A stem cell transplant is a nonsurgical alternative to a bone marrow transplant. In this procedure, which in most cases can be done on an outpatient basis and does not require general anesthesia, stem cells are removed from a woman's own bloodstream before the start of chemotherapy. They are then frozen for storage and later thawed and returned to the body through a blood transfusion. Once they are back in the body, stem cells can return to the crucial job of making blood cells and platelets. In both of these transplantation procedures, the reserved stem cells or bone marrow simply repopulate the blood cells that were destroyed by the high doses of chemotherapy drugs; they do not fight cancer.

up the medication's protective powers. Tamoxifen can prevent your cancer from returning to its original site or from escaping into the bloodstream. It may also prevent a new cancer from developing in your other breast—what doctors refer to as a contralateral breast cancer. Once you are diagnosed with breast cancer, you are three or four times more likely to become a victim of the disease again. (Even if the breast cancer that you were diagnosed with does *not* contain estrogen receptors, tamoxifen can effectively reduce your risk of contralateral disease.) Because tamoxifen works primarily by blocking the cancer-fueling effects of estrogen, it lowers recurrence and mortality rates the most in women who have cancers that are estrogen receptor positive. Studies suggest that about 65 to 80% of breast cancers in postmenopausal women contain receptors for estrogen while only about 45 to 60% of breast cancers in premenopausal women are sensitive to the stimulating effect of the hormone.

Because tamoxifen appears to fight breast cancer in a couple of ways—it does more than just interfere with estrogen's ability to bind to receptors on the surfaces of cancerous cells—the medication is not wholly without effect in women with estrogen receptor negative tumors. In these women, tamoxifen is only about 20% as effective at improving recurrence and mortality rates as it is in women with estrogen receptor positive breast cancers. Researchers are still studying the effects of using tamoxifen along with chemotherapy, although at this point it appears that a combination of the two treatments can enhance reductions in recurrence in some women with breast cancer. Studies indicate that tamoxifen is most effective when used for 5 years and that the benefits of tamoxifen therapy may last for 5 to 10 years after treatment with the medication ceases. Using the medication longer does not appear to increase your chances of staying cancer free but *does* put you more at risk for serious side effects such as endometrial cancer (cancer of the lining of the uterus) and pulmonary embolism (a blood clot in the arteries to the lungs).

Has adjuvant therapy with tamoxifen been the subject of many medical studies?

Yes. Adjuvant therapy with tamoxifen has been studied in dozens of clinical trials involving thousands of women since the medication was approved by the Food and Drug Administration (FDA) for this purpose in the mid-1980s. In 1998 adjuvant therapy with tamoxifen was the focus of a study conducted by the Early Breast Cancer Trialists' Collaborative Group (EBCTCG), which published its meta-analysis (an analysis of a number of previous medical studies) in the medical journal *Lancet*. This meta-analysis includes data from 55 clinical trials (trials that are based on actual treatment and observation of patients) of adjuvant tamoxifen involving about 37,000 women with early breast cancer. About 18,000 of the breast cancer patients included in these trials had tumors with receptors for estrogen and another 7,000 or so had breast cancers that were estrogen receptor negative. (The remaining 12,000 women included in this overview had breast cancers that were untested for the presence of estrogen receptors.) As you will see later in this chapter, the results of this meta-analysis confirm the effectiveness of tamoxifen adjuvant therapy in women who are good candidates for hormonal therapy: 20 mg a day of tamoxifen taken for 5 years results in significant improvements in recurrence and mortality rates in women with estrogen receptor positive disease and at the same time halves the likelihood of developing a contralateral breast cancer. Regardless of estrogen receptor status, 5 years of tamoxifen therapy appears to reduce the risk of developing a new breast cancer by 47% and 1 to 2 years of tamoxifen use may cut the risk by 13 to 26%.

The results of the meta-analysis indicate that the benefits of adjuvant therapy with tamoxifen are largely the same for women with breast cancer regardless of age, menopausal status, or lymph node status. Previous studies of adjuvant tamoxifen in younger women with estrogen receptor positive tumors led many researchers to believe that the medication was significantly less effective in this group of women as compared to older women with estrogen-positive cancers. Younger women have typically been treated with adjuvant chemotherapy due to a lack of evidence that tamoxifen or other hormonal therapies work as well for them. This meta-analysis provides convincing evidence that premenopausal women with estrogen-positive tumors can benefit from the use of adjuvant tamoxifen just as women in their later years do. This overview also confirms the conventional wisdom regarding tamoxifen dosage—namely that taking 30 to 40 mg a day of the medication does not offer more protection than taking only 20 mg a day.

According to this meta-analysis, which group of women benefited the most from using tamoxifen? How exactly did they benefit?

The meta-analysis clearly suggests that tamoxifen has the greatest benefit in women with estrogen receptor positive tumors who take the medication for 5 years. The higher a woman's estrogen receptor levels, the greater the benefit in terms of improved recurrence and mortality rates. For example, in the 18,000 women with breast cancers that contained estrogen receptors, the risk of recurrence was reduced as follows:

- 50% with 5 years of tamoxifen
- 28% with 2 years of tamoxifen
- 21% with 1 year of tamoxifen

Even more dramatic: In women with high levels of estrogen receptor proteins (at least 100fmol receptor per mg cytosol protein) who took tamoxifen for 5 years, the risk of recurrence was decreased by 60%. Tamoxifen was also shown to reduce mortality rates significantly in the group of women with estrogen receptor positive tumors who took the medication. The risk of death due to breast cancer was reduced as follows:

- 28% with 5 years of tamoxifen
- 18% with 2 years of tamoxifen
- 14% with 1 year of tamoxifen

In women with higher levels of estrogen receptor proteins (at least 100fmol receptor per mg cytosol protein), the risk of dying from breast cancer was reduced even further: 36% with 5 years of tamoxifen therapy. Interestingly, results from the meta-analysis suggest that mortality rates for women who took tamoxifen for 5 years continue to improve during the 5 years after treatment has stopped.

Did tamoxifen have any effect in women with estrogen receptor negative breast cancers?

Some, but the study results are not wholly clear on this point. As you saw in Chapter 5, tamoxifen does fight breast cancer in ways other than preventing estrogen from binding to cancer-cell receptors. But these alternate mechanisms of action, as they are referred to by doctors, are not very powerful and do not create significant reductions in recurrence or mortality rates. In the 7,000 or so women included in the meta-analysis whose cancers were estrogen receptor negative, the risk of recurrence was reduced as follows:

- 6% with 5 years of tamoxifen
- 13% with 2 years of tamoxifen
- 6% with 1 year of tamoxifen

As you can see, these women did receive some benefit from taking tamoxifen but the reductions are not large. If you find these statistics a little puzzling, you are not alone. It is not clear from this overview if using the medication for 5 years is any more effective than using it for 1 year in

The Benefits of Using Tamoxifen as Adjuvant Therapy

In 1998, the EBCTCG published the results of a meta-analysis involving about 37,000 women with early breast cancer who took part in clinical trials of adjuvant therapy with tamoxifen. This overview study suggests that tamoxifen greatly improves recurrence and mortality rates in women who are good candidates for hormonal therapy and also reduces the risk of new breast cancers. Women with estrogen receptor positive breast cancers who took tamoxifen for 5 years benefited the most in terms of survival and staying disease free.

Women with estrogen receptor positive tumors

- **Recurrence.** In women who took tamoxifen for 5 years, tamoxifen reduced the risk of recurrence by 50%.

- **Mortality.** In women who took tamoxifen for 5 years, tamoxifen reduced the risk of dying from breast cancer by 28%.

- **Contralateral breast cancer.** In women who took tamoxifen for 5 years, tamoxifen reduced the risk of developing a new breast cancer by 47%.

Women with estrogen receptor negative tumors

- **Recurrence.** On average, tamoxifen reduced the risk of recurrence by about 10%.

- **Mortality.** On average, tamoxifen reduced the risk of dying from breast cancer by about 6%.

- **Contralateral breast cancer.** In women who took tamoxifen for 5 years, tamoxifen reduced the risk of developing a contralateral breast cancer by 47%.

women whose breast cancers do not contain estrogen receptors. What is the explanation for this? The fact is that doctors are not certain. Further research may shed some light on the lack of a trend toward greater benefit with longer duration of tamoxifen therapy in this group of women. Tamoxifen was even less effective at improving survival rates in women with estrogen receptor negative tumors. The risk of dying from breast cancer was reduced as follows:

- 7% with 5 years of tamoxifen
- 8% with 2 years of tamoxifen
- 6% with 1 year of tamoxifen

Again, the improvements in survival are small and it is unclear whether using the medication for 5 years is any more effective than using it for 1 year in this group of breast cancer patients.

What is metastatic breast cancer?

Metastatic breast cancer occurs when cancerous cells originating in the breast invade distant parts of the body, such as the lungs or bones, by way of the bloodstream or lymphatic system. They are usually discovered as a result of symptoms or of physical exams and blood tests conducted during the periodic follow-up visits after breast cancer surgery. Keeping these appointments is crucial in order to identify a metastasis and take swift action to control it. Chest x-rays, bone scans, computed tomography (CT) scans, and magnetic resonance imaging (MRI) are also used to detect a metastasis and determine how many sites in the body are affected. The interval of time between local treatment of a breast cancer and the development of a metastasis provides an early indication of how fast the disease is moving.

Initially, most metastases involve one or two sites. The axilla (armpit), the skin and soft tissue of the chest wall, or the bones are usually affected first when a breast cancer spreads. As the disease progresses it invades other parts of the body such as the lungs or liver. The number of sites in the body affected by the metastasis, the specific areas involved, and hormone receptor status are important factors in the prognosis. Women with cancers that have metastasized to soft tissue have a more favorable outlook than those with significant bone invasion. Involvement of the central nervous system (CNS) substantially worsens the prognosis.

Tamoxifen and Endometrial Cancer

The most significant side effect reported in the EBCTCG meta-analysis is endometrial cancer. Women who took tamoxifen daily for about 5 years (the duration of therapy that is most effective at reducing recurrence and mortality rates) had a risk of developing endometrial cancer that was about four times that of women who did not take the medication. Women who used tamoxifen for 1 or 2 years had double the risk of this type of cancer. Overall, there were about 27 deaths attributed to endometrial cancer in the tamoxifen group compared to five endometrial cancer-related deaths in the group given a placebo (sugar pill). In this meta-analysis, women who took tamoxifen were no more likely than women taking placebos to die from other causes such as liver cancer, stroke (damage to part of the brain caused by lack of blood supply, due to a blockage in an artery, or the rupturing of a blood vessel), pulmonary embolism, deep vein thrombosis (a blood clot in the deep veins of the legs or pelvis), or other vascular (blood vessel) conditions. See Chapter 5 for information on the link between tamoxifen and endometrial cancer, stroke, pulmonary embolism, and deep vein thrombosis.

A metastasis to the CNS usually occurs late in the course of the disease, though in rare cases it may be one of the first sites affected. Women with metastases that are estrogen receptor positive can usually anticipate longer periods of remission and a better response (a response in this context is defined as tumor shrinkage and pain relief) not only to hormonal therapies such as tamoxifen but also to chemotherapy.

What role does tamoxifen play in the treatment of metastatic breast cancer?

Often an important one. Tamoxifen is frequently used as initial treatment in women with estrogen receptor positive cancers that do not involve vital organs and are not immediately life threatening. Tamoxifen is usually the first choice of hormonal treatment for postmenopausal women with metastatic breast cancer and has proven to be very effective in this group. Tamoxifen is used to treat metastases at a variety of sites but produces the best results in women who have bone or soft tissue involvement. Response rates are determined by hormone receptor status. About 60 to 75% of women with cancers that are estrogen receptor positive respond to therapy with tamoxifen. Postmenopausal women age 60 or over tend to benefit the most. Up to 20% of women with estrogen receptor negative cancers also experience some improvement after starting on tamoxifen. This limited efficacy may be a result of the medication's alternate mechanisms of action, which are assumed to involve growth factors (proteins that help to regulate cell growth).

How long do women with metastatic breast cancer usually take tamoxifen?

When tamoxifen is used to treat metastatic breast cancers that are estrogen receptor positive, the duration of response may last as long as 1 or 2 years. The parts of the body involved in the metastasis and levels of estrogen receptor proteins generally affect how long the benefits of tamoxifen therapy persist. Women with metastatic disease

Other Hormonal Treatments

Some women who use tamoxifen as adjuvant therapy or to treat metastatic disease develop a resistance to the medication or their breast cancers return while they are taking tamoxifen. The fact that tamoxifen therapy may become ineffective does not rule out the possibility of additional hormonal treatment in the form of medication or surgery. Women who have an initial response to tamoxifen are often good candidates for other hormonal therapies. Alternative hormonal treatments (such as those listed below) may also be used in place of tamoxifen or in women who do not have any response to the medication.

- **Progestins.** Progestins, such as medroxyprogesterone (Provera) and megestrone (Megace), are synthetic forms of progesterone, an important female sex hormone made by the ovaries that is primarily responsible for preparing the uterus for the fertilized egg and for the growth of the fetus. Progestins can block the stimulating effects of estrogen on breast cancer cells.

- **Luteinizing hormone-releasing hormone (LHRH) inhibitors.** LHRH-inhibiting medications such as goserelin (Zoladex) and leuprolide (Lupron) are used to temporarily halt the production of ovarian estrogen.

- **Aromatase inhibitors.** Aromatase inhibitors such as aminoglutethimide (Cytadren), anastrozole (Arimidex), and letrozole (Femara) reduce circulating estrogen levels by interfering with the action of the aromatase enzyme, which plays a role in the production of estrogen by the ovaries and adrenal glands.

- **Oophorectomy.** Oophorectomy is the surgical removal of the ovaries. This procedure permanently halts the production of ovarian estrogen (it does not suppress the small amount of estrogen produced in the adrenal glands), causing menopause.

Androgens. Androgens are male sex hormones. Testosterone is the primary male sex hormone, which is produced in small amounts in women. Medications such as Halotestin that contain synthetic forms of testosterone can inhibit estrogen in the breast but may cause virilization—a medical term for the development of masculine sex characteristics such as a deepening voice, hair loss, facial hair, and increased muscle mass (Halotestin may also cause acne). These side effects are usually mild and can be reversed by stopping the androgen medication or reducing dosage.

affecting bone or soft tissue often experience longer periods of remission on tamoxifen than women with metastases at other sites in the body. Tamoxifen also has more lasting effects in women whose cancers contain high levels of estrogen receptor proteins. Tamoxifen and other hormonal therapies do not produce results right away. Several months of tamoxifen therapy may be necessary before any tumor regression is detected. During the first month or so of use, many women on tamoxifen or other hormonal therapies complain of bone pain. This reaction is called a flare. It is temporary and signals that the medication is working.

Though in some cases tamoxifen may help to keep metastatic breast cancer in remission for several years, eventually most women develop a resistance to the medication. Women who stop taking tamoxifen under these circumstances may experience a phenomenon called hormonal-withdrawal response. This is a favorable reaction that can result in tumor regression for up to 6 weeks. Women who benefit from tamoxifen therapy often respond to the subsequent use of one or two additional hormonal medications. (In contrast to chemotherapy, hormonal medications are no more effective when used in combination than when used in series.) But with each additional hormonal therapy, the duration of response gets shorter. Eventually all hormonal treatments are rendered ineffective.

SEVEN

CAN TAMOXIFEN PREVENT BREAST CANCER?

QUICK FACT

In women age 35 or over who are at high risk for breast cancer, tamoxifen may reduce the likelihood of developing the disease by almost 50%.

Helen, age 38, is a lawyer who came to see me to discuss whether she should use tamoxifen (Nolvadex) to reduce the likelihood of developing breast cancer. Though premenopausal, Helen was clearly at high risk. Her two sisters were both diagnosed with the disease—one at the unusually young age of 35—and this fact alone increased Helen's risk for breast cancer by five times. Helen had also recently undergone a benign biopsy (the removal and analysis of a tissue sample) that revealed the presence of atypical hyperplasia—an excessive growth of abnormal cells that is also a breast cancer risk factor. Helen was aware of tamoxifen's performance in the Breast Cancer Prevention Trial (BCPT) and was hopeful that by using the medication she could avoid becoming the third victim in her family.

After assessing Helen's risk for breast cancer, I suggested that she consider taking a blood test for the cancer susceptibility genes BRCA1 and BRCA2. The results, I explained, might be relevant to her decision regarding whether to use tamoxifen. It is not clear from the results of the BCPT if tamoxifen has a protective effect in women who carry either of these inherited gene mutations (changes),

123

which can increase a woman's risk of developing breast cancer by 85%. The fact that Helen had multiple family members with breast cancer and a sister who got the disease at such a young age raised the specter of inherited disease. Genetic counseling helped Helen to understand the ramifications of testing for BRCA1 and BRCA2. The benefits of testing for these genes and even the accuracy of the tests themselves are a matter of controversy in the medical community. Some women decline to take the blood test because they fear if they are branded as carriers of cancer susceptibility genes they may have trouble getting health insurance or face discrimination at their jobs. Helen opted to take the blood test, the results of which indicated that she was not a carrier.

Helen, who was in good general health, also wished to discuss the most serious side effects associated with tamoxifen—endometrial cancer (cancer of the lining of the uterus) and blood clots. Her relatively young age offered her some measure of protection since both of these problems are more likely to occur in women age 50 or over who take the medication. I also explained that most women who develop this type of cancer while on tamoxifen therapy are diagnosed with early-stage disease, which can often be treated effectively. Other factors besides age affect who gets blood clots. They are more common in women who have had clots in the past or who have existing medical conditions that restrict blood flow such as diabetes, hypertension (high blood pressure), or obesity.

While not seriously overweight, Helen was about 15 pounds heavier than she should be based on her height and body type. I suggested that she start a program of proper diet and regular exercise to help shed the extra pounds. Staying fit is not only a great way to help reduce the risk of a blood clot but may also help to prevent breast cancer and a variety of other medical problems in the bargain. Once Helen felt that she understood the risks associated with tamoxifen as well as its ability to reduce the likelihood of *breast cancer, she decided to take the medication. Helen started on tamoxifen a few months after stopping her oral contraceptive (the pill) and switching to a nonhormonal form of birth control. As part of her overall preventive plan, Helen gets periodic clinical breast exams and is regularly evaluated by her gynecologist.*

It is difficult to think of another medication that has hidden such an important secret for so long—one that gives new hope to millions of American women concerned about their risk of developing breast cancer. After all, tamoxifen (Nolvadex) is one of the most well-studied anticancer drugs in the world. It has been used for over 20 years to help contain metastatic breast cancer (cancer that has spread to vital organs or bones) and since the mid-1980s to help prevent recurrence or metastasis (the spreading of cancer) after breast cancer surgery. But it was not until 1998, when doctors discovered that tamoxifen may be able to prevent breast cancer, that we began to recognize the full potential of this medication.

How did researchers arrive at this historic breakthrough in breast cancer research? Previous studies of tamoxifen had revealed clues to its possible preventive powers. When women with breast cancer took tamoxifen as adjuvant therapy (additional therapy used after primary treatment), doctors observed that their risk of developing a new breast cancer in the opposite breast (called a contralateral breast cancer) was reduced by almost *half*. If tamoxifen could prevent or delay breast cancer in these patients, might it not offer the same protection to healthy women? In 1992 researchers launched the Breast Cancer Prevention Trial (BCPT) to put tamoxifen to the test as a chemopreventive agent (a medication or other substance that has the power to prevent cancer development). One of the most important cancer prevention studies ever undertaken, the BCPT involved thousands of healthy women who were likely to develop breast cancer due to a variety of well-established risk factors. The results? Women who took tamoxifen for 5 years were nearly 50% less likely to develop breast cancer. The preliminary findings of the BCPT were so dramatic that investigators ended the study 14 months early in order to give women in the placebo (sugar pill) group a chance to benefit from tamoxifen.

It is estimated that almost 30 million women in the United States are at high risk for developing breast cancer. Most of these women rely on close monitoring of the breasts in order to detect cancer early, usually through mammography (a procedure that uses low-dose radiation to create images of the inside of the breast) and manual breast exams. Some women opt to preempt the disease at its source by undergoing prophylactic mastectomy, which involves the removal of one or both breasts before evidence of cancer is present in order to prevent the onset of the disease. Tamoxifen's newest incarnation as a potential chemopreventive promises to change the way that many women and their doctors approach the idea of preventing invasive (penetrating) disease. At the same time, it is also important to recognize that there are limitations on our knowledge of tamoxifen in its new role—we still know a lot more about tamoxifen as a treatment for breast cancer than we do about its preventive powers.

For example, we do not know for certain whether tamoxifen truly prevents breast cancer in the long run or simply delays its appearance by a few years. We also cannot rule out the possibility that some of the women in the BCPT had early, undetectable forms of breast cancer during their participation in the prevention trial. In this chapter we take a closer look at the results of the BCPT and examine the merits of tamoxifen as a risk reducer and possible chemopreventive agent. We discuss the risk criteria used in the study and explain how women who took tamoxifen benefited from the medication. This chapter also includes information on a new computer software program that can be used by you and your doctor to help assess your risk for breast cancer and to make an informed decision about using tamoxifen therapy. As you will see, the results of the BCPT also convey a powerful reminder that tamoxifen increases the risk of potentially serious and even life-threatening side effects such as uterine cancer and blood clots.

What is the BCPT?

Its full title is the National Surgical Adjuvant Breast and Bowel Project (NSABP) Breast Cancer Prevention Trial (also called NSABP Protocol P-1). It is a medical study funded by the National Cancer Institute (NCI) and designed to study the effectiveness of tamoxifen as a chemopreventive agent. In this study, which was conducted in over 300 medical centers and doctors' offices across the United States and Canada, about 13,400 women age 35 or over and at high risk for breast cancer took 20 mg of tamoxifen or a placebo daily for 5 years. To help ensure that the study was conducted without bias, it was double-blinded—meaning that neither the women who participated in the trial nor the doctors who gave them their pills were aware who received the real medication versus the placebo. The degree of breast cancer risk was calculated in several ways. Women age 60 or over were allowed to participate in the trial based on age alone. As you saw in Chapter 2, women in this age group account for over 50% of breast cancer cases in the United States each year. Women were also admitted to the study based solely on a diagnosis of lobular carcinoma in situ (LCIS). LCIS is not a true cancer but rather a marker lesion confined to the lobules (milk-producing glands). It increases by 1% per year a woman's lifetime risk for a future and more serious form of breast cancer. Women between the ages of 35 and 59 without a history of LCIS were considered for admission to the trial if they had a 5-year risk of developing breast cancer that was equal to or greater than that of women age 60 or over. Most of the women under age 60 had a combination of risk factors, which were calculated using a computer program called the Gail model. These factors include age, the number of first-degree relatives (mothers, sisters, or daughters) affected by breast cancer, a woman's age during the delivery of her first child, a history of breast biopsy (the removal and analysis of a tissue sample), a previous diagnosis of atypical hyperplasia (the excessive growth of abnormal cells), and age at onset of menstruation.

What were the results of the BCPT?

The study results, published in the *Journal of the National Cancer Institute* in 1998, suggest that tamoxifen reduces the risk of developing invasive breast cancer in high-risk women by a significant 49%. Tamoxifen also reduced the risk of noninvasive (nonpenetrating) breast cancer—such as ductal carcinoma in situ (DCIS) or LCIS—by about 50%. Women of all ages experienced these reductions in risk, which began as early as the first year of treatment

A Closer Look at the Women in the BCPT

Women young and old took part in the study. About 40% of the women in the trial were between the ages of 35 and 49, 30% were between the ages of 50 and 59, and 30% were age 60 or over. The women had a variety of risk factors, including a family history of breast cancer or a personal history of LCIS or benign (noncancerous) breast conditions. About 70% of the women in the study had at least one first-degree relative affected by breast cancer. About 6% of the women had a history of LCIS and 9% had a previous diagnosis of atypical hyperplasia. Most women who took part in the study were white. Blacks, Hispanics, and Asians (as well as other groups) made up about 4% of the study population.

with tamoxifen. The greatest protective effect was seen in women who were age 60 or over. Here are the numbers. Tamoxifen reduced the risk of breast cancer by:

- 55% in women age 60 or over
- 51% in women between the ages of 50 and 59
- 44% in women younger than age 50

Researchers also looked specifically at how the medication affected women with certain risk factors such as a history of LCIS or atypical hyperplasia. Tamoxifen reduced the likelihood of breast cancer in women with LCIS by 56% and cut the risk of the disease in women diagnosed with atypical hyperplasia by an impressive 86%.

What about women at risk for inherited breast cancer? At the moment this is a big unknown. Researchers are unable to say whether tamoxifen reduces the risk of breast cancer in women with BRCA1 or BRCA2 gene mutations (changes) because these genes were only identified after the BCPT began. Doctors are now analyzing blood samples taken from women who participated in the trial in order to determine if tamoxifen has any protective effect in women who carry these cancer susceptibility genes. In addition to its effects on breast cancer risk, tamoxifen also had bone-building benefits. The risk of fractures in the wrist, hip, and spine—the most common sites of osteoporotic fractures—was reduced by almost 20% in women taking tamoxifen. Though tamoxifen is known to reduce cholesterol levels in some women, there is no difference to date in the number of heart attacks between the tamoxifen group and those women taking placebo.

What does the BCPT show?

It is important to be clear on this point. The BCPT indicates that tamoxifen reduces the risk of breast cancer development in women at high risk who take the medication for 5 years. That much doctors can agree on. Anything further that we extrapolate from the findings of the BCPT is a matter of speculation, no matter how well-informed. The Food and Drug Administration (FDA) approved tamoxifen as a risk reducer but has not sanctioned the belief that tamoxifen actually *prevents* breast cancer from developing in the long run or that it works in women at low-to-moderate risk for the disease. Why the uncertainty? We do not know at this point whether taking tamoxifen for 5 years only delays the appearance of cancer because long-term studies are not complete. The question of whether tamoxifen is truly a chemopreventive agent will have to wait until we have monitored the progress of women in the BCPT and in other studies for about 10 or 15 years. It is even possible that some of the women in the BCPT *already had* very early forms of breast cancer and that tamoxifen was being used to combat existing disease in such cases. As you saw in Chapter 6, breast cancer cells can occur in such tiny amounts that they are undetectable by any available methods.

Do we have any clues as to whether tamoxifen's possible preventive effects last? We may. A number of medical studies have established tamoxifen's ability to reduce the risk of new breast cancers in women who take the medication as adjuvant therapy. Tamoxifen has been shown to reduce the likelihood of such contralateral breast cancers by 47%—this figure is reassuringly similar to the almost 50% reductions in risk observed in the BCPT—and its protective effects appear to last in the long term. It is therefore reasonable to speculate that tamoxifen's preventive effects in healthy women at high risk may also persist for a decade or longer. We will know a lot more about tamoxifen's powers as a possible chemopreventive after the year 2002 when we can observe the medication's long-term protective effects in the early participants of the BCPT.

Did women who took tamoxifen in the BCPT experience side effects?

Yes. These side effects ranged from merely bothersome to deadly. Hot flashes and vaginal discharge were the most frequent complaints. Other common side effects associated with tamoxifen, which are described in Chapter 5, were also reported. The most serious problems affected the older women in the study. These include endometrial cancer (cancer of the lining of the uterus), pulmonary embolism (a blood clot in the arteries to the lungs), and deep vein thrombosis (a blood clot in the deep veins of the legs or pelvis). Tamoxifen doubled the risk of endometrial cancer and tripled the likelihood of developing pulmonary embolism. These potentially life-threatening medical problems occurred more often in women age 50 or over. The younger women in the study did not experience a significant increase in the risk of these side effects. Tamoxifen did not appear to increase the likelihood of any cancer other than uterine. See Chapter 5 for more information about the link between tamoxifen and endometrial cancer, pulmonary embolism, and deep vein thrombosis.

- **Endometrial cancer.** The increased risk for endometrial cancer was seen mainly in women age 50 or over who took tamoxifen. They were four times more likely to develop endometrial cancer than were women who took placebo. Overall, there were 36 cases of endometrial cancer in the tamoxifen group versus 15 cases in the placebo group. All endometrial cancers diagnosed in women taking tamoxifen were early, stage 1 forms of the disease. Most caused abnormal vaginal bleeding or pain as a symptom.

- **Pulmonary embolism.** This side effect caused fatalities. Three women in the tamoxifen group who developed pulmonary embolism died as a result of the problem. Overall there were 18 cases of pulmonary embolism in the tamoxifen group as opposed to six cases in the placebo group.

- **Deep vein thrombosis.** The risk for this vascular (blood vessel) disorder was increased by over 50% in the tamoxifen group. There were 35 cases of deep vein thrombosis in the tamoxifen group versus 22 cases in the placebo group.

- **Cataracts.** Tamoxifen slightly increased the risk of developing cataracts (a clouding of the lens of the eye) and of the need for surgery to correct the problem.

What is the Breast Cancer Risk Assessment Tool?

The Breast Cancer Risk Assessment Tool (BCRAT)—also called the risk disk—is a computer software program available at no cost from the NCI that can help you and your doctor assess your risk for breast cancer. It was developed by researchers at the NCI and NSABP in 1998 for use on Macintosh or IBM PC computers. The BCRAT can be used to evaluate a number of risk factors in order to compute your 5-year and lifetime breast cancer risk and to help determine whether or not you would benefit from starting on preventive therapy with tamoxifen. The BCRAT can compare your breast cancer risk to that of a woman your age who has no major risk factors and also to the risk levels of women in the BCPT.

The risk assessment software program may not be helpful to every woman who is concerned about her risk for breast cancer. It cannot be used to reliably estimate the risk of women younger than age 20, women who have already been diagnosed with breast cancer, or women who have breast cancer susceptibility genes such as BRCA1 or BRCA2. A more refined version of the risk assessment software program is in development for release to the public in early 1999. This version aims at computing hypothetical, individualized outcomes for women who are considering tamoxifen therapy and wish to know beforehand what sort of risk reduction they can expect with the medication.

What are some of the reasons that women may not be able to use tamoxifen?

That is a good question. It is important to understand that the BCRAT is not designed to do your thinking for you

How Many Women Will Be Able to Use Tamoxifen to Reduce Their Risk?

It is estimated that almost 30 million women in the United States may be eligible to take tamoxifen to help reduce their risk of breast cancer development. This number includes all women age 60 or over, all women age 35 or over with LCIS, and other women between the ages of 35 and 59 who have high-risk profiles. (The following percentages are based strictly on risk and do not take into account other factors, such as pregnancy or a history of blood clots, that may prevent women from taking tamoxifen.)

Age	Percentage of American women in this age group who may be good candidates for tamoxifen
35	0.3
40	2.7
45	7.1
50	9.3
55	12.5
60 or over	100

Note: This last statistic is easy to misinterpret. Though all women age 60 or over are at high risk for breast cancer based on age, tamoxifen is not the right choice for *all* women in this age group. See below for more information on why some women are not able to take the medication.

Source: Adapted from the National Cancer Institute.

or to make decisions that only you can and should make about your health. The choice of whether or not to use tamoxifen as a risk reducer is a personal decision that you must make in conjunction with your doctor, who is your expert partner in the process. The risk assessment software program can be useful in helping you weigh the potential benefits of using tamoxifen against the risk of potentially serious side effects such as endometrial cancer or pulmonary embolism. Some women at increased risk for breast cancer may not be good candidates for tamoxifen therapy due to such factors as existing medical conditions, the use of oral contraceptives (the pill) or postmenopausal estrogen therapy, or an existing or planned pregnancy. For example, women at increased risk of blood clots may not be able to take tamoxifen because it increases the risk of vascular problems. Blood clots tend to occur more often in older women or women who have hypertension (high blood pressure) or diabetes. The risk of serious blood clots is also higher in women who smoke or are obese.

Women who take oral contraceptives or use estrogen therapy in the form of estrogen replacement therapy (ERT) or hormone replacement therapy (HRT)—which is a combination of estrogen and progesterone—cannot take tamoxifen. Combining tamoxifen with hormone-containing contraceptives or medication may cause unwanted and potentially dangerous effects. (In addition, oral contraceptives as well as ERT and HRT may be a contributing factor in the development of breast cancer.) Women who take oral contraceptives or use estrogen therapy must stop taking these medications several months before starting on tamoxifen. Women who are pregnant or plan to get pregnant within the next several years cannot take tamoxifen because animal studies suggest that it may harm the fetus (developing baby).

What sorts of factors are evaluated using the BCRAT?

The BCRAT evaluates several major risk factors for breast cancer. These factors, which are listed below, include age, a family history of breast cancer, a diagnosis of noninvasive breast cancer, age during delivery of a first child, age at onset of menstruation, a history of breast biopsy, and race. You may notice that some of the risk factors discussed in Chapter 2 are not taken into account by the BCRAT. There are two reasons for this. The risk assessment software program is designed to evaluate well-established variables that represent a fairly precise degree of risk. It is true that there are a variety of other factors that may increase the risk of breast cancer as well. These include age at menopause, the use of hormone-containing contraceptives or postmenopausal estrogen therapy, a high-fat diet, and alcohol intake, to name a few. But the risk associated with some of these factors is difficult to quantify (in other words, doctors cannot assign to them a number that accurately represents the risk increase they pose) and other factors are as yet unproven.

- **Age.** Besides being female, age is the single biggest risk factor for breast cancer development. In fact, about 77% of women diagnosed with breast cancer are over age 50. As you saw earlier in this chapter, if you are age 60 or over you may be able to take tamoxifen even if you have no other risk factors.

- **Family history of breast cancer.** Your risk for breast cancer rises depending on the number of first-degree relatives you have who are affected by the disease. Having one first-degree relative affected by breast cancer doubles your risk, while having two first-degree relatives with the disease increases your risk by five times.

- **Noninvasive breast cancer.** The presence of LCIS increases by 1% a year your risk for developing invasive breast cancer in the future.

- **Age during delivery of your first child.** A woman who is age 30 or over during the delivery of her first-born is more at risk of developing breast cancer than a woman who gives birth earlier in life. Studies suggest that if you had your first child after age 30, you have a twofold to fivefold increase in risk compared to a woman who first gave birth before age 18 or 19. Women who have never given birth are also more at risk.

- **Onset of menstruation.** If you started menstruation early (before age 12), this elevates your lifetime exposure to estrogen and therefore slightly increases your risk for breast cancer.

- **Breast biopsy.** A history of breast biopsy is associated with an increased risk for breast cancer (this is not a result of the biopsy procedure itself). In particular, a diagnosis of atypical hyperplasia increases your risk.

- **Race.** White women are slightly more at risk of developing the disease than are black women or women of other ethnic groups.

Is it true there are two other studies of tamoxifen that suggest it does *not* reduce the risk of breast cancer?

True. Is this another case of mixed messages echoing from different quarters of the halls of medical science? Probably not—more like comparing apples and oranges. Let us survey what we know about these clinical trials—one is Italian and the other British—and explain how they are different from the BCPT. The results of the foreign studies, both of which were designed to test tamoxifen as a chemopreventive agent, were published in the *Lancet* in 1998. In both studies, there was no significant difference in breast cancer incidence between women taking tamoxifen and women who took placebo. How to explain this? Differences in what doctors call study design may provide the answers as to why tamoxifen turned out to be a dud in the two foreign studies and an effective risk reducer in the BCPT. For one thing, the two European studies involved smaller study populations—about 4,500 women in the Italian trial and slightly more than half that number in the study conducted in the United Kingdom. When it comes to clinical trials—particularly prevention trials—bigger is usually better. All things being equal, larger studies tend to reveal outcomes more clearly and reliably than trials involving fewer participants. The BCPT involved more than 13,400 women.

There are other important differences as well. The Italian and British trials used risk criteria different from that of the BCPT. The Italian study involved postmenopausal women between the ages of 35 and 70 who had a low-to-normal risk of breast cancer development. The BCPT only admitted women at high risk for the disease. The British study involved women between the ages of 30 and 70 who had an increased risk of developing breast cancer based on a sole risk factor: a family history of the disease. This means that the trial in the United Kingdom may have inadvertently recruited large numbers of women who carry breast cancer susceptibility genes such as BRCA1 or BRCA2. As you saw earlier in this chapter, it is unknown if tamoxifen therapy is effective in reducing the risk of breast cancer in women with these inherited gene mutations.

The use of postmenopausal estrogen therapy by study participants is another major difference between the European studies and the BCPT. Some of the women in the two foreign studies were on estrogen therapy while they took tamoxifen. Estrogen-containing medications such as ERT or HRT may interfere with the ability of tamoxifen to bind with estrogen receptors and produce its protective effects. (In addition, many doctors believe that ERT and HRT actually increase the risk of developing breast cancer.) The bottom line? Most doctors do not believe that the two European studies discredit the findings of the BCPT.

Are You a Good Candidate for Tamoxifen Therapy?

This book cannot evaluate your personal risk for breast cancer. But it may be helpful to examine some of the high-risk profiles listed below—which are provided by the NCI—to get a sense of how combinations of risk factors in women of certain ages can affect the likelihood of breast cancer. Keep in mind that you may be at high risk even if your profile does not match any of those listed below. Women age 60 or over or who have LCIS are considered potential candidates for therapy with tamoxifen in the absence of any other risk factors.

If you are age 35, you may be able to take tamoxifen if your risk profile resembles one of the following scenarios:

- **Scenario 1.** You have a first-degree relative affected by breast cancer, a history of two or more benign biopsies, and a previous diagnosis of atypical hyperplasia.

- **Scenario 2.** You have a first-degree relative affected by breast cancer, a history of two or more benign biopsies, you were age 25 or over during the delivery of your first child, and you began menstruating before age 12.

- **Scenario 3.** You have two first-degree relatives affected by breast cancer and a history of at least one breast biopsy.

If you are age 40, you may be able to take tamoxifen if your risk profile resembles one of the following scenarios:

- **Scenario 1.** You have two first-degree relatives affected by breast cancer and you were age 29 or over during the delivery of your first child.

- **Scenario 2.** You have two first-degree relatives affected by breast cancer and you are childless.

- **Scenario 3.** You have a first-degree relative affected by breast cancer and a previous diagnosis of atypical hyperplasia.

If you are age 45, you may be able to take tamoxifen if your risk profile resembles one of the following scenarios:

- **Scenario 1.** You have two first-degree relatives affected by breast cancer.

- **Scenario 2.** You have a first-degree relative affected by breast cancer and you started menstruating before age 12.

- **Scenario 3.** You have a first-degree relative affected by breast cancer and a history of at least one breast biopsy.

If you are age 50, you may be able to take tamoxifen if your risk profile resembles one of the following scenarios:

- **Scenario 1.** You have a first-degree relative affected by breast cancer and you were age 20 or over during the delivery of your first child.

- **Scenario 2.** You have a previous diagnosis of atypical hyperplasia and you were age 20 or over during the delivery of your first child.

- **Scenario 3.** You have a previous diagnosis of atypical hyperplasia and are childless.

- **Scenario 4.** You have a previous diagnosis of atypical hyperplasia and you started menstruating before age 12.

If you are age 55, you may be able to take tamoxifen if your risk profile resembles one of the following scenarios:

- **Scenario 1.** You have a first-degree relative affected by breast cancer.

- **Scenario 2.** You started menstruating before age 12 and you were age 30 or over during the delivery of your first child.

- **Scenario 3.** You have a previous diagnosis of atypical hyperplasia.

EIGHT

TAMOXIFEN AND THE SEARCH FOR A WONDER DRUG: SELECTIVE ESTROGEN RECEPTOR MODULATORS AND PURE ANTIESTROGENS

QUICK FACT

In addition to being an effective anti-cancer medication, tamoxifen can strengthen bones and reduce levels of fat in the bloodstream.

Joanne, age 55, is a postmenopausal flight instructor who went to a local endocrinologist in order to discuss preventive therapy for osteoporosis—an age-related, gradual weakening of the bones. Her mother had recently broken her hip—a common site of osteoporotic fracture—after a slight fall. It was a serious injury requiring several months of rehabilitation. Knowing that osteoporosis runs in families, Joanne became concerned about her bone health. Dual energy x-ray absorptiometry (DEXA)—a noninvasive (non-penetrating) procedure that uses low-dose radiation to evaluate the strength of the bones—revealed that Joanne had dangerously weak bones and was at increased risk for a fracture. Joanne and her doctor had discussed what she could do to reduce her risk of developing osteoporosis. The preventive strategy they crafted together included calcium supplements and a program of regular, weight-bearing exercise. Joanne had also discussed with her doctor the possibility of starting on hormone replacement therapy

(HRT)—a combination of estrogen and progesterone—but was concerned about the increased risk for breast cancer associated with supplemental estrogen medications. Joanne's doctor suggested a bone-building agent called raloxifene (Evista), a relatively new selective estrogen receptor modulator (SERM). Joanne was especially interested to learn that raloxifene may have the additional benefit of reducing breast cancer risk. She wanted to discuss this aspect of the medication—as well as her risk for breast cancer—with an oncologist (a doctor who specializes in the treatment of cancer) so her doctor referred her to me.

Joanne and I assessed her risk for breast cancer and discussed possible ways for her to maintain healthy breasts while increasing the strength of her bones. I explained that while Joanne did not have a high-risk profile at the time of our conversation, in a few years her likelihood of developing breast cancer would increase based on her age alone. Joanne was aware that tamoxifen (Nolvadex) has bone-building effects in addition to being an effective anticancer medication and wondered if using tamoxifen after she turned 60 was a good way to keep her bones strong and possibly help to prevent breast cancer. I explained to Joanne that tamoxifen was not recommended as long-term, preventive therapy for osteoporosis because it increases the risk of endometrial cancer and other serious medical problems. As Joanne's endocrinologist had explained, maintaining adequate bone strength may require the use of a bone-building medication for a decade or longer. As a proven osteoporosis medication and possible chemopreventive agent (a medication or other substance that has the power to prevent cancer development), raloxifene was a better choice for Joanne. It is not linked with an increased risk of endometrial cancer and may even help to prevent the disease by blocking the effects of estrogen in the uterus. I also told Joanne that the medication may reduce her risk of breast cancer by 50 to 70% and lower her total cholesterol and high density lipoprotein (LDL) cholesterol levels. After weighing the potential benefits of raloxifene against its risks—the most serious being an increased risk of blood clots—Joanne decided to start taking 60 mg a day of raloxifene. Joanne has been taking raloxifene for 2 years now. Her bones have gotten stronger and she remains cancer free.

Unlike local treatment for breast cancer, which often consists of surgery and radiation therapy designed to eliminate cancerous cells from the breast, tamoxifen (Nolvadex) is a systemic (whole body) therapy. It roams freely through the bloodstream, acting like estrogen in some parts of the body while blocking the hormone's effects in others—what doctors refer to as a selective estrogen receptor modulator (SERM). By inhibiting estrogen in breast cancer cells that have hormone receptors, tamoxifen starves the disease of the hormonal fuel it needs to thrive. By acting like estrogen in other areas of the body, such as the skeleton and cardiovascular system, tamoxifen may help to prevent osteoporosis (an age-related, gradual weakening of the bones) and heart disease. Both are serious medical conditions that women tend to experience after menopause when they lose the protection provided by estrogen. While studies suggest that tamoxifen strengthens bones and helps to keep blood vessels healthy, the medication is not prescribed as preventive therapy for osteoporosis or heart disease because it can cause serious side effects such as endometrial cancer (cancer of the lining of the uterus) and other health problems.

Doctors are also studying other medications with antiestrogenic (estrogen-blocking) effects—some of these medications are SERMs while others are pure antiestrogens—as treatments for breast cancer or as chemopreventive agents (medications or other substances that have the power to prevent cancer development). Raloxifene is a bone-building SERM medication for postmenopausal women that may have beneficial effects on the cardiovascular system and also reduce the risk of breast cancer development. Unlike tamoxifen, raloxifene does not appear to stimulate the uterus and is not associated with an increased risk of endometrial cancer. Because of raloxifene's effects on the skeleton and blood vessels, the medication is used by some women as an alternative to estrogen therapy after menopause. Despite the benefits of estrogen therapy, many women choose not to use it for fear that it may cause breast or uterine cancer or other unwanted side effects.

Toremifene (Fareston) is another new SERM. Used to treat metastatic breast cancer (a cancer that has spread to vital organs or bones) in postmenopausal women, toremifene is an effective alternative to tamoxifen when used as first-line hormonal therapy for advanced forms of the disease. Doctors are also studying antiestrogens such as ICI 182, 780 (Faslodex). ICI 182, 780 and other antiestrogens lack the dual hormonal nature of SERMs. They are designed only as estrogen blockers and do not have estrogen-like effects in any part of the body. Still under study, ICI 182, 780 appears to be effective when used as additional hormonal therapy for women who develop a resistance to tamoxifen.

Do women really need to be concerned about heart disease?

Absolutely. No postmenopausal woman can afford to take her cardiovascular health for granted. It may surprise you to learn that heart disease is the number one killer of American women, claiming the lives of 500,000 women each year. Half of those deaths are due to heart attacks. (By comparison, breast cancer is responsible for the deaths of almost 44,000 women annually.) Taking steps to keep your heart healthy is important at every age but this is especially true as you get older. It is after menopause that a woman's ovaries stop producing the estrogen critical to protecting the cardiovascular system from diseases such as coronary heart disease (CHD), the type of heart disease that can lead to a heart attack. In CHD, an artery supplying the heart with blood becomes thickened and hardened due to the buildup of cholesterol and other substances on the artery wall. When this plaque, as it is called, partially or totally blocks the flow of blood, the heart may be deprived of the oxygen it requires to pump effectively (blood clots that form on the surface of plaque can also obstruct blood flow). This can result in a heart attack, in which areas of the heart actually die because they are starved for oxygen. Within a decade after menopause, women experience heart attacks at about the same rate as men. Eating a low-fat diet and getting regular exercise in your younger years can help to protect your cardiovascular system from disease in the decades after menopause.

Is it true that tamoxifen can lower cholesterol levels?

Yes. Tamoxifen's estrogenlike effects in cardiovascular tissue can lower levels of fats in the blood that affect your risk for heart disease. Studies suggest that tamoxifen reduces total blood cholesterol levels by 12% and levels of

---

How Estrogen Helps to Keep the Heart Healthy

Estrogen plays an important role in maintaining the health of the cardiovascular system by delivering chemical "messages" that have an effect on the tissue in that area. It does this by connecting to hormone receptors in the arteries where plaque tends to accumulate. These receptors, which are like communication ports, are located on the surfaces of cells. It is believed that estrogen boosts the effectiveness of the healthier fats in the bloodstream and helps to prevent the buildup of plaque on artery walls. Estrogen may also aid in the washing away of fatty deposits by increasing the flow of blood.

low density lipoprotein (LDL) cholesterol—also called bad cholesterol—by 20% (see below for more information about bad cholesterol). These reductions may help to prevent CHD and heart attack in women who use the medication. In a clinical trial called the Scottish Adjuvant Tamoxifen Trial, there was a 63% reduction in heart attack deaths in women taking tamoxifen. Measurements of total blood cholesterol and LDL cholesterol are important because they reflect the health of the heart and blood vessels. Cholesterol is a waxy, fatty substance produced by the body and also found in foods that come from animals. In high amounts it can contribute to the buildup of plaque in the arteries. High levels of total blood cholesterol are associated with an increased risk for heart disease. Before menopause, most women have healthy total cholesterol levels— a desirable number is under 200 mg/dL. These levels tend to increase as women age. A woman between the ages of 45 and 64, for example, is likely to have a total cholesterol level in the range of 217 to 237 mg/dL.

Doctors also measure LDL cholesterol to evaluate heart disease risk. Lipoproteins are cholesterol-hauling proteins. Cholesterol, which does not dissolve in the blood, is transported through the body by LDL or high-density lipoprotein (HDL). LDL cholesterol and HDL cholesterol differ from one another in terms of the amount of fat they carry and where they deposit their cholesterol cargo. LDL cholesterol hauls the most fat and releases it directly onto the lining of your arteries, where it may build up and form plaque. This explains why it is referred to as bad cholesterol and why it is desirable to have less of it in your body—a desirable level being below 130 mg/dL. HDL cholesterol is the "alter ego" of LDL cholesterol. Known as the good cholesterol, it carries its smaller cargo of fat *away* from the arteries and deposits it in the liver. There cholesterol is passed from the body or used to make other necessary and healthier substances. When it comes to HDL cholesterol, a higher number is better than a lower number. Once your HDL cholesterol level falls below 35 mg/dL, your risk of heart disease begins to climb. While tamoxifen can lower levels of total cholesterol and LDL cholesterol, it does not have an effect on HDL levels.

Is it true that tamoxifen can help to strengthen bones?

Yes and no. Tamoxifen has the power to strengthen or weaken bones depending on whether or not the woman taking it has completed menopause. Studies indicate that in postmenopausal women tamoxifen can preserve or increase bone density (the amount of mineral in any given volume of bone), particularly in the spine. But in premenopausal women tamoxifen can actually cause a loss of bone strength. While tamoxifen's bone-weakening effects in younger women are not fully understood, doctors believe that in postmenopausal women the medication has an estrogenlike effect on bone.

The complex, dynamic process referred to as bone remodeling is important to understanding how tamoxifen helps to preserve bone strength in older women. The key players in this process are the mineral calcium and bone cells called osteoclasts and osteoblasts. Calcium, as most women know, is a building block of bone. Osteoclasts and osteoblasts are involved in the process by which bones grow stronger and denser or become weaker and brittle. The osteoclast group of cells dismantles bone. Their job is to remove the building blocks of calcium and other minerals from your bones—essentially removing bone, bit by bit—and send them back into the bloodstream. The osteoblast cells form a tiny construction crew. While the osteoclasts are removing small bits of bone, the osteoblasts are busy filling in the holes with calcium and other minerals that they remove from the bloodstream. Whichever type of cell is able to do its job better—the osteoclasts that destroy bone or the osteoblasts that build bone—determines the health of your bones at any stage in your life. So where does tamoxifen enter the picture? By acting like estrogen in the skeleton, tamoxifen tips the scales in this contest between bone cells. Tamoxifen chemically encourages the osteoblasts to work harder, stimulates the activity of vitamin D (vitamin D facilities the body's absorption of calcium from food), and has effects on other hormones that influence bone remodeling.

Is osteoporosis a major problem for postmenopausal women?

Very much so. This gradual weakening of the bones due to loss of estrogen after menopause has reached almost epidemic proportions in the United States. Osteoporosis affects over 28 million Americans according to the National Osteoporosis Foundation (NOF)—and 90% of them are postmenopausal women over age 50. The disease causes a loss of bone density that results in lighter, more porous bones. This means that the bones are less capable of bearing normal weight and break much more easily. Because osteoporosis is a silent disease and typically causes no symptoms, the first indication of it is often a fracture. A woman with osteoporosis can experience a fracture as a result of a slight fall, lifting a bag of groceries, or even after stepping off a curb. The bones of the hip, spine, and wrist are particularly vulnerable. Many women are unaware of the consequences that a hip fracture can have on their overall health. Though a hip fracture itself is not immediately life threatening, about 20% of women who suffer this type of injury die within 6 months, and 10 to 20% die within a year. The mortality rates associated with hip fractures occur largely because fractures of this sort often result in complications such as blood clots, stroke, pneumonia, and other serious conditions. The good news is that osteoporosis can usually be prevented with a calcium-rich diet, weight-bearing exercise, and medication (when necessary).

What is raloxifene?

Raloxifene is a SERM approved by the Food and Drug Administration (FDA) in 1997 for preventing and treating osteoporosis in postmenopausal women. It is a powerful bone-builder that appears to have a healthy effect on the cardiovascular system by reducing blood fat levels. In 24-month osteoporosis prevention trials, raloxifene lowered total blood cholesterol by about 5% and LDL cholesterol by about 8%. Like tamoxifen, raloxifene does not appear to affect levels of HDL cholesterol. Studies are ongoing to determine whether raloxifene reduces heart attack risk in postmenopausal women who take the medication. What excites some women most about raloxifene is its potential as a chemopreventive agent. Short-term studies suggest that raloxifene blocks the effects of estrogen in the breast and may help to reduce the risk of breast cancer by 50 to 70% in women who have completed menopause. Unlike tamoxifen, raloxifene does *not* appear to act like an estrogen in the uterus and has not been linked to an increase in endometrial cancer.

In the Multiple Outcomes of Raloxifene Evaluation (MORE) trial, 7,700 postmenopausal women under age 80 who had osteoporosis were given raloxifene (60 or 120 mg) or placebo. The MORE trial, a double-blind study conducted in 180 sites around the world, was designed to test whether raloxifene reduces the risk of fractures. Investigators also sought to determine if raloxifene reduces the risk of breast and endometrial cancer. In this study, about 3 years of raloxifene reduced the risk of breast cancer by about 70% and appeared to reduce the risk of endometrial cancer as well—regardless of whether women took 60 mg or 120 mg dosages of the medication. Raloxifene is also being tested in clinical trials as a treatment for metastatic breast cancer.

I've heard that there is another breast cancer prevention trial underway that compares tamoxifen to

raloxifene. Can you tell me more about this?

In this large-scale clinical trial, the two medications will go head-to-head as risk reducers. The Study of Tamoxifen and Raloxifene (STAR) is scheduled to open at 400 sites across the United States and Canada in early 1999, pending approval by the FDA. Also referred to as the National Surgical Adjuvant Breast and Bowel Project (NSABP) Protocol P-2, the trial will involve 22,000 healthy, postmenopausal women at increased risk for developing breast cancer. While the final inclusion criteria for the trial are not yet decided, it is expected that women participating in STAR must be age 35 or over and postmenopausal and must be at high risk for breast cancer based on factors such as age, the number of first-degree relatives (mothers, sisters, or daughters) with the disease, a history of benign (noncancerous) breast biopsy (the removal and analysis of a tissue sample), age during delivery of a first child, and age at onset of menstruation. Women who participate in STAR will randomly receive either 20 mg of tamoxifen or 60 mg of raloxifene daily for 5 years. Unlike most clinical trials, which test a medication by comparing it to a placebo, the STAR trial will test one established risk reducer (tamoxifen) against another possible chemopreventive agent (raloxifene). You can contact the NSABP for more information about the trial. See the Resources section at the end of this book for contact information for the NSABP.

What about other SERMs?

Toremifene, developed in a Finnish laboratory in the late 1970s, was approved by the FDA in 1997 for the treatment of metastatic breast cancer in women who have completed menopause. It is mainly used as an alternative to tamoxifen as hormonal therapy in women with estrogen receptor positive cancers. In some studies, 60 mg of toremifene has produced response rates (a response in this context is tumor shrinkage and pain relief) of 48 to 68% in women with metastatic breast cancer. Because toremifene appears to

Medications with Antiestrogenic Effects

- **Tamoxifen.** As you have seen earlier in this book, this SERM is used to treat breast cancer in all its forms and is proven to reduce the likelihood of breast cancer development in women at high risk. It strengthens bone and lowers levels of important fats in the blood. Tamoxifen also acts like estrogen in the uterus, increasing the risk of endometrial cancer.

- **Raloxifene.** This SERM is an osteoporosis medication for postmenopausal women. It helps to keep the cardiovascular system healthy by reducing blood fat levels. Short-term studies suggest that raloxifene may also be a potent chemopreventive agent, reducing breast cancer risk by up to 70%. It does not appear to stimulate the tissue of the uterus and may even reduce the likelihood of endometrial cancer.

- **Toremifene.** Toremifene is a SERM that resembles and is cross-resistant with tamoxifen. It can be used to treat metastatic breast cancer in postmenopausal women and has bone-building effects as well. The medication lowers total blood cholesterol and LDL cholesterol levels while increasing levels of HDL cholesterol.

- **ICI 182, 780.** A pure antiestrogen, ICI 182, 780 does not have estrogenlike effects in any part of the body. Still under study, this medication may one day be used as additional hormonal therapy for women who develop a resistance to tamoxifen. ICI 182, 780 may also prove to be an effective first choice for adjuvant therapy after breast cancer surgery.

work by binding to estrogen receptors on the surfaces of breast cancer cells, it is most effective in women whose cancers test positive for hormone receptors. Toremifene appears to be "cross-resistant" with tamoxifen. This means that toremifene has little or no benefit for women who have been previously treated with tamoxifen. Because of this cross-resistance, toremifene is typically given to women with advanced forms of breast cancer who have not been treated previously with hormonal therapy. Besides strengthening bones, toremifene outshines tamoxifen and other SERMs when it comes to improving blood fat levels. Toremifene not only lowers total blood cholesterol and LDL cholesterol levels but increases heart-friendly HDL cholesterol. Unfor-tunately, toremifene also acts like estrogen in the uterus. This means that it stimulates the tissue there and may cause an increased risk of endometrial cancer. Though toremifene is only approved for treating metastatic breast cancer, it may have potential as adjuvant therapy (additional therapy used after primary treatment) or as a chemopreventive medication.

How are SERMs different from antiestrogens? Are there any important antiestrogens on the horizon?

While SERMs have the ability to block the effects of estrogen in some tissues and mimic its effects in others, pure antiestrogens lack this hormonal split personality. They travel through the bloodstream and block the effects of the hormone in all parts of the body—breast, uterus, bone, blood vessels, and elsewhere. Antiestrogens were first developed by researchers at Zeneca pharmaceuticals, the company that manufactures tamoxifen. The most intriguing antiestrogen to emerge so far is ICI 182, 780. Still in the research stage, this medication appears to be effective when used to treat women who have experienced recurrences of breast cancer while on tamoxifen or who develop tamoxifen-dependent tumors (masses of abnormal cells that may be either cancerous or benign). In one clinical trial, ICI 182,

780 was given as a monthly injection to 19 women with metastatic breast cancer who developed a resistance to tamoxifen. The medication produced responses in 69% of the women and continued to work for an average of 2 years. Most women in the study reported minimal side effects (headache was the most common complaint). Because ICI 182, 780 combats breast cancer cells by starving them of the hormonal fuel they need to grow, ICI 182, 780 has no effect against breast cancers that lack estrogen receptors. Though more study is needed, antiestrogens such as ICI 182, 780 may become powerful weapons in the fight against advanced forms of breast cancer. The catch? Because ICI 182, 780 also blocks the effects of estrogen in the bones and cardiovascular system, it may contribute to the development of osteoporosis or heart disease.

APPENDIX A: RESOURCES

Stay Informed

Taking an active role in your breast health involves educating yourself about breast cancer and the therapies used to treat or prevent it. Once you become accustomed to the idea of looking for health information, you may be surprised at the number of available resources. Information on breast cancer and medications such as tamoxifen (Nolvadex) can be found in books, medical journals, educational materials provided by health organizations, patient education brochures, newspapers, on television and radio programs, and on the Internet. The more you learn about breast cancer, the easier it is to evaluate what you read and hear and avoid information overload. For a start, get into the habit of reading a major newspaper or news magazine or watching the news on TV. These days, developments in the world of medicine—such as the results of major medical studies—often grab headlines. Many newspapers have sections dedicated to health issues and TV programs often feature medical correspondents who provide regular reports on health news. While health-related information that appears in the media is often sensationalized or poorly analyzed, newspapers and TV programs can often alert you to breast cancer studies that you may wish to ask your doctor about or investigate more thoroughly on your own.

There are several national health organizations, such as the National Cancer Institute (NCI) and the American Cancer Society (ACS), that provide free or low-cost educational materials relating to breast cancer. You can access these materials by contacting the organizations or visiting their Web sites. Support groups are another excellent way to stay informed. Sharing information with other women who have breast cancer or who are at high risk for the disease can help identify the best doctors in your area and shed light on what treatments work best. Many women also find that talking to other breast cancer survivors helps them to cope with the emotional consequences of a cancer diagnosis. Local support groups can often be located by contacting organizations such as the NCI or ACS. You may also be able to find support groups in your community by calling the major medical centers or university hospitals near you. See below for contact information for the NCI and ACS.

The Internet

Not an expert Web surfer? No problem. You do not need to be a frequent flyer in cyberspace to learn the basics of information gathering on the Internet. Search engines, such as Metacrawler, Altavista, Excite, WebCrawler, and Yahoo, make it easy to do Internet searches on specific topics. All you need are a few keywords to start exploring this vast online resource. Once in a search engine, you can use search words such as "breast cancer" or "tamoxifen" to find relevant Web sites. Most of the organizations listed below have Web sites on the Internet as well. The NCI and ACS Web pages are great places to start. Medline is a cost-free, searchable database containing thousands of medical journal abstracts. Many Web sites on the Internet post health-related information and often provide links to other areas of interest including online support groups. Online sites can also provide a network of support and encouragement in the form of newsgroups and chat rooms. Newsgroups are areas in which people provide information and answer questions.

In a chat room, you can participate in a real-time, ongoing group conversation on just about any subject. But no matter where your virtual travels take you on the Web, caution is key when using the Internet as a source of medical information. While many legitimate organizations post information on the Web, there are no guarantees that all the facts and recommendations that you find there are sound. It is also common to encounter a few well-disguised sales pitches. The rule: Always discuss medical information that you discover on the Internet with your doctor. See below for contact information for the NCI, ACS, and Medline.

Locating an FDA-Certified Mammography Facility in Your Area

There are several ways to go about finding a certified facility near you. If you have access to the Internet, you can visit the Web site of the Food and Drug Administration (FDA) and download a free listing of FDA-certified mammography (a procedure that uses low-dose radiation to create images of the inside of the breast) centers located across the country. You can also contact the ACS or the Mammography Information Service of the NCI for information on how to find a mammography center in your area that meets federal guidelines. You can buy a computer disk containing a list of federally approved facilities in the United States by calling the National Technical Information Service (NTIS). You can buy a single disk or a subscription—the subscription entitles you to four updated disks a year. It is important to keep in mind that the certification status of a mammography center can change. This means that the FDA-approved facility you visited last year to get your mammogram (an x-ray of the breast) may no longer meet federal guidelines 1 or 2 years later. Always check the FDA certification status of your mammography center before getting a mammogram there. See Chapter 2 for more information on how to get the best mammogram. See below for contact information for the FDA, NCI, ACS, and NTIS.

Organizations that Provide Information or Support

African American Breast Cancer Alliance
2265 Como Avenue, Suite 10
St Paul, MN 55108
Phone: (612) 644-1224

American Association for Cancer Research
6th & Chestnut, Public Ledger 816
Philadelphia, PA 19106
Phone: (215) 440-9300
http://www.aacr.org

American Cancer Society
1599 Clifton Road NE
Atlanta, GA 30329
Phone: (800) ACS-2345
http://www.cancer.org/cancinfo.html

American College of Obstetricians and Gynecologists
Office of Public Information
409 12th Street Southwest
Washington, DC 20024
Phone: (202) 484-3321
http://www.acog.com

American College of Radiology
1891 Preston White Drive
Preston, VA 22091
Phone: (800) 227-5463
http://www.acr.org

American Heart Association
7272 Greenville Avenue
Dallas, TX 75231
Phone: (800) AHA-USA1
http://www.amhrt.org

American Institute for Cancer Research
1759 R Street NW
Washington, DC 20009
Phone: (800) 843-8114
http://www.aicr.org

American Medical Association
515 North State Street
Chicago, IL 60610
Phone: (312) 464-4818
http://www.ama-assn.org

American Medical Women's Association
801 North Fairfax Street, Suite 400
Alexandria, VA 22314
Phone: (703) 838-0500
http://www.amwa-doc.org/index.html

American Society of Clinical Oncology
750 17th Street NW, #1100
Washington, DC 20006
Phone: (703) 299-0150
http://www.asco.org

American Society of Cytopathology
400 West 9th Street, Suite 201
Wilmington, DE 19801
Phone: (302) 429-8802
Fax: (302) 429-8807
http://www.cytopathology.org

American Society of Plastic and Reconstructive Surgeons
444 East Algonquin Road
Arlington Heights, IL 60005
Phone: (708) 228-9900
Referral message tape: (800) 635-0635
http://www.plasticsurgery.org

American Society of Therapeutic Radiation/Oncology
1891 Preston White Drive
Reston, VA 22091
Phone: (703) 648-3794

Avon's Breast Cancer Awareness Crusade
http://www.avoncrusade.com

Beth Israel Health Care System's Guide to Breast Cancer
http://www.bimc.edu:80/netscape2/breastcancer/intro.html

Bone Marrow Transplant Family Support Network
PO Box 845
Avon, CT 06001
Phone: (800) 826-9376

Breast Cancer Action Group
PO Box 5605
Burlington, VT 05402
Phone: (802) 863-3507

Breast Cancer Action
55 New Montgomery, Suite 323
San Francisco, CA 94105
Phone: (415) 243-9301
Fax: (415) 243-3996
http://www.bcaction.org/index.html

Breast Cancer Advisory Center
PO Box 224
Kensington, MD 20895
Phone: (301) 949-1132

Breast Cancer Information Clearinghouse
http://nysernet.org/bcic

Breast Cancer Support Program
Adelphi University
School of Social Work
PO Box 703
Garden City, NY 11530
Phone: (516) 877-4320

Breast Health Institute
1015 Chestnut St, Suite 510
Philadelphia, PA 19107-4305
Phone: (215) 627-4447
http://www.breast-health.org

Breast Implant Information Foundation
177 Willow Street
Lockport, NY 14094
Phone: (716) 433-6432

Breast Implant Support
101118 Daisy Avenue
Palm Beach Gardens, FL 33410
Phone: (407) 622-5469

Cancer Care Inc.
1180 Avenue of the Americas, 2nd floor
New York, NY 10036
Phone: (800) 813-HOPE
http://www.cancercareinc.org

Cancer Prevention Coalition
520 N Michigan Avenue, Suite 410
Chicago, IL 60611
Phone: (312) 467-0800
Fax: (312) 467-0599

Centers for Disease Control and Prevention
1600 Clifton Road NE
Atlanta, GA 30333
Phone: (404) 639-3311
http://www.cdc.gov

CHEMOcare
231 N Avenue
Westfield, NJ 07090
Phone: (908) 233-1133 or (800) 55-CHEMO
http://nysernet.org/bcic/numbers/chemo.html

Chemotherapy Foundation
183 Madison Avenue, Suite 403
New York, NY 10016
Phone: (212) 213-9292

Community Breast Health Project at Stanford University
http://www-med.stanford.edu:80/cbhp

Empowering Younger Women with Breast Cancer
University of Wisconsin Women's Clinic
6630 University Avenue
Middleton, WI 53562
Phone: (608) 263-7527

Endometriosis Association
8585 N 76th Place
Milwaukee, WI 53223
Phone: (414) 355-2200
http://www.endometriosisassn.org

Food and Drug Administration
5600 Fisher's Lane
Rockville, MD 20857
Phone: (301) 827-2410
http://www.fda.gov

**Food and Drug Administration Breast Implant
Information Hotline**
Phone: (800) 532-4440

Harvard Health Publications
*http://www.countway.harvard.edu/publications/Health_
Publications/home.html*

Healthfinder
http://www.healthfinder.org/default.htm

Linda Creed Breast Cancer Foundation
Medical Tower Building
255 South 17th Street, Suite 905
Philadelphia, PA 19103
Phone: (215) 545-0800
Fax: (215) 545-8503
http://www.libertynet.org/~lcbcf/art.html

LymphEdema Foundation
PO Box 834
San Diego, CA 92014-0834
Phone: (800) LYMPH-DX
http://lymphedemafoundation.org

Mary Helen Mautner Project for Lesbians with Cancer
1707 L Street NW, Suite 1060
Washington, DC 20036
Phone: (202) 332-5536
http://www.mautnerproject.org

Mayo Health Oasis
http://www.mayohealth.org/mayo/common/htm/index.htm

MEDLINE
http://www.nlm.nih.gov/databases/freemedl.html

Memorial Sloan-Kettering Guttman Diagnostic Center
55 Fifth Avenue, 12th Floor
New York, NY 10003
Phone: (212) 463-8733
http://www.mskcc.org/document/pedgutmn.htm

Menopause News
2074 Union Street
San Francisco, CA 94123
Phone: (800) 241-MENO
http://www.well.com/user/mnews/html/experts.htm

Menopause Online
http://www.menopause-online.com

Mothers Supporting Daughters with Breast Cancer
c/o Charmayne Dierker
21710 Bayshore Rd
Chestertown, MD 21260-4401
Phone: (410) 778-1982
http://www.azstarnet.com/~pud/msdbc/index.html

National Alliance of Breast Cancer Organizations
9 E 37th Street, 10th Floor
New York, NY 10016
Phone: (800) 719-9154
http://www.nabco.org

National Bone Marrow Donor Program
3433 Broadway St NE, Suite 400
Minneapolis, MN 55413
Phone: (800) 654-1247
http://www.marrow.org

National Bone Marrow Transplant Link
29209 Northwestern Highway #624
Southfield, MI 48034
Phone: (800) LINK-BMT
http://www.comnet.org/nbmtlink

National Breast Cancer Coalition
1707 L Street NW, Suite 1060
Washington, DC 20036
Phone: (202) 296-7477
Fax: (202) 265-6854
http://www.natlbcc.org

National Cancer Institute
31 Center Drive, MSC 2580
Bethesda, MD 20892-2580
Phone: (800) 4-CANCER
http://www.nci.nih.gov

National Coalition for Cancer Survivorship
1010 Wayne Avenue, 5th Floor
Silver Spring, MD 20910
Phone: (301) 650-8868
http://www.cansearch.org

National Foundation for Cancer Research
7315 Wisconsin Avenue, Suite 500
Bethesda, MD 20814
Phone: (301) 654-1250
http://www.nfcr.org

National Health Information Center
U. S. Department of Health and Human Services
PO Box 1133
Washington, DC 20013
Phone: (301) 565-4167 or (800) 336-4797
http://www.nhic-nt.health.org

National Institute on Aging
PO Box 8057
Gaithersburg, MD 20898
Phone: (800) 222-2225
http://www.nih.gov/nia

National Lymphedema Network
2215 Post Street, Suite 404
San Francisco, CA 94115
Phone: (800) 541-3259
http://www.lymphnet.org

National Osteoporosis Foundation
1150 17th Street NW, Suite 500
Washington, DC 20036
Phone: (202) 223-2226
http://www.nof.org

National Surgical Adjuvant Breast and Bowel Project
East Commons Professional Building
Four Allegheny Center, 5th floor
Pittsburgh, PA 15212-5234
Phone: (412) 330-4600
Fax: (412) 330-4660
http://www.nsabp.pitt.edu

National Technical Information Service
Technology Administration
US Department of Commerce
Springfield, VA 22161
Phone: (703) 605-6000
Fax: (703) 605-6900
http://www.ntis.gov

National Women's Health Resource Center
5255 Loughboro Road NW
Washington, DC 20016
Phone: (202) 537-4015
http://www.healthywomen.org/about.html

National Women's Health Network
514 10th Street NW, Suite 400
Washington, DC 20004
Phone: (202) 344-1140
http://www.aoa.dhhs.gov/aoa/dir/203.html

North American Menopause Society
University Hospitals
Department of Ob/Gyn
PO Box 94527
Cleveland, OH 44101
Phone: (216) 844-8748
http://www.menopause.org

OncoLink
http://cancer.med.upenn.edu

Oncology Nursing Society
501 Holiday Drive
Pittsburgh, PA 15220
Phone: (412) 921-7373
http://www.ons.org

Patient Advocates for Advanced Cancer Treatments
1143 Parmelee NW
Grand Rapids, MI 40504
Phone: (616) 453-1477
http://www.osz.com/paact

Radiation Therapy Oncology Group
1101 Market Street, 14th Floor
Philadelphia, PA 19107
Phone: (215) 574-3191
http://www.rtog.org

Silicone Disease Network
186 Lions Gate Drive
Columbia, SC 29223
Phone: (803) 699-5037

Sisters Network, National Headquarters
8787 Woodway Drive, Suite 4207
Houston, TX 77063
Phone: (713) 781-0255
Fax: (713) 780-8998
http://www.users.aol.com/sistersnet/sis.html

Society of Gynecologic Oncologists
401 N Michigan Avenue
Chicago, IL 60611-4267
Phone: (312) 644-6610
http://www.sgo.org

Society of Surgical Oncology
85 W Algonquin Road, #550
Arlington Hts, IL 60005-4425
Phone: (847) 427-1400

Susan G. Komen Foundation
Occidental Tower
5005 LBJ Freeway, Suite 370
Dallas, TX 75244
Phone: (800) IM-AWARE
http://www.komen.org

Virginia Breast Cancer Foundation
5001 W Broad Street, #28
PO Box 17884
Richmond, VA 23226
Phone: (800) 345-VBCF
http://www.medhlp.netusa.net/agsg/agsg463.htm

Wellness Community
2716 Ocean Park Boulevard, Suite 1040
Santa Monica, CA 90504
Phone: (310) 314-2555
http://www.wellnesscommunity.org

Women's Cancer Network
2413 W River Road
Grand Island, NY 14072
Phone: (800) 562-2623
http://www.wcn.org

World Health Organization
Regional Office for the Americas
Pan American Health Organization
525 23rd Street NW
Washington, DC 20037
Phone: (202) 974-3000
http://www.who.org

Y-Me Breast Cancer Organization
212 W Van Buren Street, 5th Floor
Chicago, IL 60607-3908
Phone: (800) 221-2141
http://www.y-me.org

Zeneca Pharmaceuticals
1800 Concord Pike
Wilmington, DE 19850
Phone: (302) 886-3000
Fax: (302) 886-2972
http://www.usa.zeneca.com

Organizations that Provide Information Mainly on Alternative Therapies

The American Association of Naturopathic Physicians
PO Box 20386
Seattle, WA 98102
Phone: (206) 323-7610
http://www.naturopathic.org

The American Holistic Medical Association
4101 Lake Boone Trail, #201
Raleigh, NC 26707
Phone: (919) 787-5146
http://www.ahmaholistic.com

The Herb Research Foundation
1007 Pearl Street, Suite 200
Boulder, CO 80302
Phone: (303) 449-2265
http://www.herbs.org/index.html

National Center for Homeopathy
801 N Fairfax Street, Suite 306
Alexandria, VA 22314
Phone: (703) 548-7790
http://www.healthy.net/pan/pa/homeopathic/natcenhom

Books on Breast Cancer and Tamoxifen

Arnot R. B., Arnot B. *Breast Cancer Prevention Diet: The Powerful Foods, Supplements, and Drugs that Can Save Your Life.* Boston: Little Brown, 1998.

Bazell R., Bernstein A. *Her-2: The Making of Herceptin, a Revolutionary Treatment for Breast Cancer.* New York: Random House, 1998.

Berger K, Bostwick J. *A Woman's Decision: Breast Care, Treatment and Reconstruction.* New York: Tor, 1998.

Brinker N. G., McEvilly Harris, C. *The Race Is Run One Step at a Time: Every Woman's Guide to Taking Charge of Breast Cancer & My Personal Story.* Indianapolis: Summit, 1995.

Casten L. C. *Breast Cancer: Poisons, Profits & Prevention.* Monroe, ME: Common Courage, 1997.

Chronicle Books Staff. *Art, Rage, Us: Art and Writing by Women with Breast Cancer.* San Francisco: Chronicle, 1998.

Dackman L. *Affirmations, Meditations, and Encouragements for Women Living with Breast Cancer.* Upland, PA: DIANE, 1998.

Davies K., White M. *Breakthrough: The Race to Find The Breast Cancer Gene.* New York: John Wiley & Sons, 1996.

Degregorio M. W., Wiebe V. J. *Tamoxifen and Breast Cancer.* New Haven, CT: Yale, 1994.

Diamond H. *You Can Prevent Breast Cancer.* San Diego: ProMotion Publishing, 1996.

Dunnavant S., Wilson, N. *Celebrating Life: African American Women Speak out about Breast Cancer.* Dallas: Usfi, 1995.

Eckmann J. K. *Breast Cancer: Strategies for Husbands to Support Their Wives.* Nehemiah, 1995.

Eisenpreis B. *Coping: A Young Woman's Guide to Breast Cancer Prevention.* New York: Rosen, 1996.

Epstein S., LeVert S., Steinman D. *The Breast Cancer Prevention Program.* New York: Macmillan General Reference, 1998.

Falcone R. *Natural Medicine for Breast Cancer.* New York: Dell, 1997.

Feldman G. *You Don't Have to Be Your Mother.* New York: WW Norton, 1995.

Fore R. C., Fore R. E. *Survivors' Guide to Breast Cancer: A Couple's Story of Faith, Hope, and Love.* Macon, GA: Smyth and Helwys, 1998.

Friedeberger J. *A Visible Wound: A Healing Journey through Breast Cancer.* Boston: Element, 1996.

Gabbard A. *No Mountain Too High: A Triumph over Breast Cancer; The Story of the Women of Expedition Inspiration.* Seattle: Seal Press Feminist, 1998.

Gale A. H. *Older than My Mother: A Nurse's Life & Triumph over Breast Cancer.* Seattle: Ananse, 1996.

Gelmon K. *Breast Cancer: All You Need to Know to Take an Active Part in Your Treatment.* Intelligent Patient Guide, 1998.

Goodson-Kjome P. *This Adventure Called Life: Healing From Breast Cancer Naturally.* New York: Sunshine, 1995.

Grigg M. L. *Breast Cancer and You: Bettering the Odds.* Brookline Village, MA: Branden, 1995.

Hirshaut Y., Pressman P. I. *Breast Cancer: The Complete Guide.* New York: Bantam, 1996.

Honea C. H. *The First Year of the Rest of Your Life: Reflections for Survivors of Breast Cancer.* Cleveland, OH: Pilgrim, 1997.

Hunter M. A. *The Little Book of Breast Cancer: A Self-Teaching Guide.* CancerInfo, 1998.

Jordan V. C. *Tamoxifen: A Guide for Clinicians & Patients.* Publisher Research and Representation, 1997.

Joseph B., Herman P. *My Healing from Breast Cancer.* New Canaan, CT: Keats, 1996.

Keon J. *The Truth about Breast Cancer: A 7-Step Prevention Plan.* Parissound, 1998.

Kneece J. C. *Finding a Lump in Your Breast: Where to Go… What to Do.* Seattle: Edu Care, 1996.

Kneece J. C. *Helping Your Mate Face Breast Cancer: Tips for Becoming an Effective Support Person for the One You Love during the Breast Cancer Experience.* Seattle: Edu Care, 1995.

Kneece J. C. *Your Breast Cancer Treatment Handbook: Your Guide to Understanding the Disease, Treatments, Emotions and Recovery from Breast Cancer.* Seattle: Edu Care, 1998.

Lange V. *Be a Survivor: Your Guide to Breast Cancer Treatment.* Hollywood, CA: Lange, 1998.

Lauersen N. H., Stukane E. *The Complete Book of Breast Care.* New York: Fawcett, 1998.

Love, S. *Dr. Susan Love's Breast Book.* Reading, MA: Perseus, 1995.

Mayer M., Lamb L. *Advanced Breast Cancer: A Guide to Living with Metastatic Disease.* Sebastopol, CA: O'Reilly, 1998.

Mayer M., Lamb L. *Holding Tight, Letting Go: Living with Metastatic Breast Cancer.* Sebastopol, CA: O'Reilly, 1997.

McCarthy P. *Breast Cancer?: Let Me Check My Schedule!* Boulder, CO: Westview, 1997.

Michnovicz J. J., Klein D. S. *How to Reduce Your Risk of Breast Cancer.* New York: Warner, 1996.

Moody M. R. *Breast Cancer Sisters.* Many Hearts, 1998.

Moody M. R., Schockney L. *Courage and Cancer: A Breast Cancer Diary—A Journey from Cancer to Cure.* Gardiner, NY: Rhache, 1996.

Moss S. *Keep Your Breasts: Preventing Breast Cancer the Natural Way.* Source, 1998.

Olmstead L. *Breast Cancer and Me: A Humorous Hope-Filled Story of a Breast Cancer Survivor.* Camp Hill, PA: Christian, 1996.

Phelan McCoy L., Keitlen T., Swearenger M. *Twenty Something & Breast Cancer: Images in Healing.* In Print, 1995.

Phillips R. H., Goldstein P. *Coping With Breast Cancer.* Wayne, NJ: Avery, 1998.

Pike J. *A Safe Place: A Journal for Women Diagnosed with Breast Cancer.* Custer, WA: Orca, 1997.

Ploski C. *Conversations with My Healers: My Journey to Wellness from Breast Cancer.* Tulsa, OK: Council Oak Distribution, 1997.

Porter M. E. *Hope Is Contagious: The Breast Cancer Treatment Survival Handbook.* New York: Fireside, 1997.

Rinzler C. A. *Estrogen and Breast Cancer: A Warning to Women.* Alameda, CA: Hunter House, 1996.

Rosenthal M. S. *The Breast Sourcebook: Everything You Need to Know About Cancer Detection, Treatment and Prevention.* Los Angeles: Lowell House, 1997.

Sherrill M. S. *Portraits of Hope: Conquering Breast Cancer: 52 Inspirational Stories of Strength.* New York: Stewart Tabori and Chang, 1998.

Shockney L. *Breast Cancer Survivors' Club: A Nurse's Experience.* Port St. Lucie, FL: Windsor House, 1997.

Singletary S. E. *Breast Cancer.* New York: Springer-Verlag, 1999.

Sokol B., Falkenberry J. *Breast Cancer: A Husband's Story.* Birmingham, AL: Crane Hill, 1997.

Springer M. *A Tribe of Warrior Women: Breast Cancer Survivors.* Birmingham, AL: Crane Hill, 1996.

Stabiner K. *To Dance with the Devil: The New War on Breast Cancer.* New York: Dell, 1998.

Swirsky J. *The Breast Cancer Handbook: Taking Control after You've Found a Lump.* New York: Harper Perennial, 1998.

Wadler J. *My Breast: One Woman's Cancer Story.* New York: Pocket, 1997.

Weed S. S. *Breast Cancer, Breast Health: The Wise Woman Way.* Saugerties, NY: Ash Tree, 1996.

Weiss M. C. *Living beyond Breast Cancer: A Guide for Survivors for when Treatment Ends and the Rest of Your Life Begins.* New York: Times, 1998.

Wooddell M. J., Hess D. J. *Choosing Alternative and Complementary Therapies.* New York: New York University, 1998.

GLOSSARY

adjuvant therapy: additional therapy used after primary treatment.

adrenal glands: glands located near the kidneys that produce hormones regulating metabolism and blood pressure; the adrenal glands produce a small amount of estrogen, even after menopause.

aerobic exercise: exercise that helps to condition the heart and lungs by making them work harder to meet the increased oxygen demands of the body.

alveoli: tiny sacs within the lobules in the breast that produce and store milk.

ampullae: see milk reservoirs.

androgen: an important male sex hormone found in small amounts in women.

aneuploid cells: cells that contain an abnormal amount of material in their nuclei.

angina: chronic condition characterized by brief episodes of chest pain or shortness of breath.

areola: the darker-hued, circular patch of skin that surrounds the nipple.

atherosclerosis: hardening of the arteries.

atypia: the presence of abnormal cells.

atypical hyperplasia: an excessive growth of abnormal cells.

173

axilla: the medical term for the armpit.

axillary dissection: a surgical procedure that involves the removal of the axillary lymph nodes adjacent to the affected breast in order to determine if a breast cancer has metastasized to the lymph nodes and how many are affected.

axillary lymph nodes: lymph nodes located under the arm; most of the fluid collected by lymph vessels in the breast is filtered by axillary lymph nodes.

benign: noncancerous.

biochemical marker: a substance found in blood or urine that gives doctors clues to processes going on inside the body.

biopsy: the removal and analysis of a tissue sample.

bone density test: a medical test used to estimate the strength of the bones.

bone density: the amount of mineral in any given volume of bone.

bone remodeling: the process by which bones are broken down (by osteoclast cells) and rebuilt (by osteoblast cells) over a lifetime.

breast-conserving surgery: any procedure that involves the removal of a cancerous tumor from the breast along with a portion of breast tissue; also called breast-sparing surgery.

breast-sparing surgery: see breast-conserving surgery.

calcium: a mineral that acts as an important building block of bone and is used by the body for proper functioning of organs and muscles.

cancer: an unrestrained growth of abnormal cells, often in the form of a tumor, that invades and destroys healthy tissue.

cancer susceptibility gene: an inherited gene mutation that greatly increases the risk of developing certain types of cancer.

capillaries: the smallest blood vessels.

carcinoma: a type of cancer that arises in epithelial tissue.

cardiovascular system: the system responsible for circulating blood throughout the body; it is composed mainly of the heart and blood vessels.

cataracts: a clouding of the lens of the eye.

chemopreventive agent: a medication or other substance that has the power to prevent cancer development.

chemotherapy: the use of certain medications to treat infections or cancer.

cholestasis: the failure of the liver to produce amounts of bile sufficient for proper digestion.

cholesterol: a soft, fatty substance made by the body and also found in foods that come from animals.

colloid carcinoma: see mucinous carcinoma.

contralateral breast cancer: the development of a new breast cancer that appears in the opposite breast of a woman who has already been diagnosed with the disease.

core needle biopsy: a nonsurgical technique that involves using a needle about $1/16$ in. in diameter and $1/2$ in. long to withdraw a cylinder of tissue from a breast abnormality.

cyst: a fluid-filled cavity.

cytopathologist: a doctor who analyzes cell samples.

diploid cells: cells that contain a normal amount of genetic material in their nuclei.

duct ectasia: a hard lump under the areola that results from a clogged milk duct.

ductal carcinoma in situ (DCIS): a cancer that is confined to its original site in a milk duct; also called noninvasive ductal carcinoma or intraductal carcinoma.

early breast cancer: a cancer that is confined to the breast or that has metastasized only as far as the axillary lymph nodes.

early menopause: menopause that occurs before age 40.

edema: swelling, usually in the legs and ankles but sometimes in other parts of the body as well, due to fluid retention.

endocrine system: a complex biological network composed of organs and glands that secrete hormones to other areas of the body in order to regulate reproduction and growth, digestion, bone building, calorie burning, body temperature, and metabolism.

endometrial cancer: cancer of the lining of the uterus.

epithelial tissue: the tissue found on the surfaces of the body such as the skin or the internal linings of organs or glands.

estradiol: the main estrogen; produced by the ovaries, estradiol operates from puberty to menopause and is measured by doctors to determine estrogen levels.

estrogen receptors: proteins on the surfaces of cells that bind with estrogen.

estrogen replacement therapy (ERT): the use of an estrogenlike medication to replace estrogen lost due to menopause.

estrogen: the primary female sex hormone; estrogen, which is primarily made by the ovaries until menopause, can fuel the growth of certain breast cancers.

Evista: see raloxifene.

excisional biopsy: a surgical procedure that involves the removal an entire lump or mass; it is the most invasive type of biopsy procedure and provides the most information about a breast abnormality.

fat necrosis: a solid lump of damaged fatty tissue that usually forms at the site of a bruise or surgical incision.

fetus: a developing baby.

fibroadenoma: the most common type of solid, benign lump found in the breast; fibroadenomas can be as small as peas or as large as oranges and usually strike women in their late teens or early 20s.

fibrocystic changes: the lumpiness or breast pain that most women experience during the 2 weeks or so before a menstrual period.

fine needle aspiration (FNA): a nonsurgical technique that involves the insertion of a very thin needle (thinner than a needle used to draw blood) through the skin and into a cyst in order to draw fluid from it, which causes it to collapse.

fine needle aspiration biopsy (FNAB): a nonsurgical technique that involves the insertion of a very thin needle (thinner than a needle used to draw blood) through the skin and into a breast abnormality in order to withdraw cell samples for the purpose of analysis.

fracture: a break in a bone.

gland: a cell (or group of cells) or an organ that produces substances (such as hormones) used by the body.

growth factor: a type of protein that helps to regulate cell growth.

heart attack: a degeneration of the heart muscle that results from inadequate blood supply to the area.

hepatitis: liver inflammation.

hepatic necrosis: the death of liver tissue.

high-density lipoprotein (HDL): a protein that tends to carry cholesterol away from the arteries and back to the liver, where it is passed from the body or used to make other substances; also called good cholesterol.

hormone: a chemical message carrier produced by an organ or gland that travels through the bloodstream to specific receptors located on the cells of other organs or glands (a hormone fits into a cell receptor the way a key fits into a lock) where it either turns on or turns off—or speeds up or slows down—activity at the site.

hormone receptor status test: a test that determines whether or not breast cancer cells contain receptors for estrogen or other hormones; the presence of receptors indicates that estrogen may be fueling the cancer's growth.

hormone replacement therapy (HRT): the use of a medication that combines progesterone and estrogen.

hot flash: a sudden rush of warmth, lasting anywhere from several seconds to several minutes and varying in intensity, that starts in the chest and radiates into the neck and face.

hydrogenated fat: fat that has undergone a process that causes it to become more saturated; hydrogenated fat is found in many margarine products and in some prepared foods.

hyperplasia: an excessive growth of cells.

hypothalamus: the part of the brain above the pituitary gland that regulates many body functions such as body temperature, sleep, and appetite.

hysterectomy: the surgical removal of the uterus.

in situ: literally, in position; an in situ breast cancer is one that is confined to a duct or lobule.

incisional biopsy: an outdated surgical procedure that involves removing a portion of a tumor by making an incision in the breast.

inflammatory breast cancer: a rare, aggressive, quickly spreading carcinoma that causes the breast to appear red, warm, and swollen.

insulin-like growth factor (IGF): a growth factor that accelerates cell proliferation.

intraductal carcinoma: see ductal carcinoma in situ.

intraductal papilloma: a small, warty growth occurring under the areola that is difficult to palpate but may cause pain or a bloody discharge from the nipple.

invasive breast cancer: a cancer that has spread from its original site in a duct or lobule and invaded surrounding breast tissue and possibly other parts of the body.

lipoprotein: a type of protein that transports fats in the blood.

lobe: one of 15 to 20 clusters of lobules contained in each breast.

lobular carcinoma in situ (LCIS): a marker lesion that indicates an increased risk of developing breast cancer in either breast at some point in the future; also called non-invasive lobular carcinoma.

lobule: a milk-producing gland of the breast.

low-density lipoprotein (LDL): a protein that tends to deposit cholesterol onto the walls of the arteries, where it may build up and form plaque; also called bad cholesterol.

lumpectomy: a breast-conserving surgical procedure that involves the removal of a cancerous tumor and a few centimeters of surrounding, cancer-free tissue.

lymph nodes: small filtering units (ranging in size from a pinhead to a bean) located in clusters in different parts of the body that neutralize the bacteria, toxins, and cell debris that circulate between cells.

lymph vessels: tiny tubes, branching into all the tissues of the body, that collect the fluid circulating between cells and transport it to the lymph nodes for filtering.

lymphatic system: a system of organs and tissues that is vital to the body's ability to fight infection and disease.

lymphedema: a swelling of the arm due to a buildup of lymphatic fluid that cannot drain in the absence of the axillary lymph nodes; it is a complication associated with axillary dissection.

mammogram: an x-ray of the breast.

mammography: a procedure that uses low-dose radiation to create images of the inside of the breast.

mastectomy: the removal of one or both breasts.

mechanism of action: the process or processes by which a medication produces its effects.

medullary carcinoma: type of invasive breast cancer, accounting for about 5% of all breast cancer cases, that has well-defined margins between the tumor and disease-free, surrounding breast tissue.

menopause: the day on which menstrual periods have stopped for a period of 1 year, occurring around age 50; this term is also used to refer to the entire process during which the ovaries slow down and finally cease producing estrogen.

metastasis: the spread of cancer.

metastatic breast cancer: a cancer that has metastasized to vital organs or bones.

microcalcifications: tiny calcium deposits that usually indicate a benign condition but are sometimes cancerous.

milk duct: one of the transport tubes designed to carry breast milk from the lobules to the nipple pores.

milk reservoir: one of the temporary holding tanks (which are actually just widened areas of ducts located near the nipple) that are the last stop for breast milk before it is expelled through the nipple pores.

modified radical mastectomy: a surgical procedure that involves the removal of the entire breast along with one or more lymph nodes.

monounsaturated fat: a type of unsaturated fat.

mucinous carcinoma: a type of invasive breast cancer characterized by a slow growing mass of mucus-producing cancer cells; also called colloid.

multicentric breast cancer: a cancer that is located in more than one quadrant of the breast.

multifocal breast cancer: a cancer that is located in more than one position but still within a limited portion of the breast.

mutation: change.

natural killer cells: a specialized, elite core of white blood cells that is marshaled by the immune system to attack tumors or viruses.

night sweats: hot flashes that occur at night during sleep.

nipple pores: exit passages located in the nipple through which milk is expelled from the breast.

node-negative breast cancer: a cancer that has not metastasized to the axillary lymph nodes.

node-positive breast cancer: a cancer that has metastasized at least as far as the axillary lymph nodes.

Nolvadex: see tamoxifen.

noninvasive: nonpenetrating.

noninvasive breast cancer: a cancer that is confined to its original site in a duct or lobule.

noninvasive ductal carninoma: see ductal carcinoma in situ.

noninvasive lobular carcinoma: see lobular carcinoma in situ.

nuclear grade: a number from 1 to 3, rating the ability of cancer cells to divide and grow, that helps to distinguish slower-growing from more aggressive tumors.

oncogene: a gene associated with the healthy, controlled growth of cells.

oncologist: a doctor who specializes in the treatment of cancer.

oophorectomy: the surgical removal of the ovaries.

ophthalmologist: a doctor who treats diseases of the eye.

osteoclasts: the cells that remove calcium and other minerals from bone and send them back into the blood, making bone weaker.

osteoporosis: an age-related, gradual weakening of the bones that causes them to become more fragile and vulnerable to potentially debilitating fractures.

ovary: the female reproductive organ that produces eggs. The ovaries are where most estrogen is made in women.

Paget's disease: A rare form of breast cancer that affects the nipple and areola and is usually associated with an underlying carcinoma.

palpate: feel.

partial mastectomy: a breast-conserving surgical procedure that involves removing a portion of breast tissue.

pathologist: a doctor who conducts microscopic analysis of tissue samples.

pectoral muscles: the wall of muscle that separates the breast from the ribcage.

perimenopause: the several years leading up to menopause; most women enter perimenopause in their late 30s or early 40s.

placebo: a sugar pill; a placebo is used mainly in controlled experiments to test the efficacy of another substance (usually a medication).

plaque: a buildup of cholesterol and other substances in the lining of an artery.

ploidy: the amount of genetic material in the nucleus of a cell.

polyp: a growth originating in a mucous membrane that is usually benign but can be cancerous.

polyunsaturated fat: a type of unsaturated fat.

postmenopausal: a term referring to a woman who has completed menopause.

progesterone: an important female sex hormone made by the ovaries that is primarily responsible for preparing the uterus for the fertilized egg and for the growth of the fetus.

progestin: a synthetic form of progesterone.

prognosis: the outlook for recovery.

prognostic factors: factors that affect prognosis.

prophylactic mastectomy: the removal of one or both breasts before evidence of cancer is present in order to prevent the onset of the disease.

protein: a substance, made up of amino acids, which helps to grow and repair tissue in the body and also forms the basis for new bone.

pulmonary embolism: a blood clot in the arteries to the lungs.

quadrantectomy: a breast-conserving surgical procedure similar to a lumpectomy except that it removes more tissue—about 25% of the breast.

radiation: a type of energy found in x-rays and ultraviolet light.

radiation therapy: the use of a beam of radiation, targeted at certain areas of the breast, to kill any cancerous cells that may remain in the breast or nearby tissues after a lumpectomy or other breast-conserving surgery.

radical mastectomy: an outdated surgical procedure that involves the removal the entire breast, the pectoral muscles that lie behind it, and one or more lymph nodes.

radiologist: a doctor trained in the interpretation of x-ray and other images.

raloxifene: a bone-building medication approved by the Food and Drug Administration (FDA) in 1997 for osteoporosis; the trade name for raloxifene is Evista.

retinopathy: one of several disorders of the retina.

risk factor: anything that makes you more likely to develop a disease.

sarcoma: a tumor that arises in connective tissue or bone.

saturated fat: a type of fat, found mainly in foods that come from animals and in certain vegetable oils, that can raise your blood cholesterol levels.

selective estrogen receptor modulator (SERM): a type of medication that mimics the effects of estrogen in certain parts of the body while blocking its effects in others.

sentinel node biopsy: a new type of surgical procedure, involving the injection of a radioactive substance or a blue dye into a cancer and the removal of the first axillary lymph node that receives it, used to sample axillary lymph nodes for the presence of cancerous cells.

simple mastectomy: a surgical procedure that involves the removal of the entire breast but leaves the lymph nodes in place.

sonogram: an image produced by sound waves.

sonography: the use of high-frequency sound waves to create an image of the inside of the body.

s-phase fraction: a number assigned to a tumor that indicates its growth rate and reflects the percentage of cancerous cells that are in the process of dividing.

stroke: damage to part of the brain caused by lack of blood supply (due to a blockage in an artery) or the rupturing of a blood vessel.

surgical menopause: an onset of menopause caused by the surgical removal of the ovaries.

systemic: whole body.

tamoxifen: a medication that can be used to treat all stages of breast cancer and that reduces the risk of breast cancer development in healthy women at high risk; the trade name of tamoxifen is Nolvadex.

testosterone: a male sex hormone produced in the testes.

thrombosis: a blood clot.

TNM system: an objective set of criteria used by doctors to measure the extent of a breast cancer and to help determine further treatment.

transforming growth factor (TGF) alpha: a growth factor that accelerates cell proliferation.

transforming growth factor (TGF) beta: a growth factor that inhibits cell proliferation.

tubular carcinoma: a type of invasive breast cancer, resembling the tubelike shape of a duct, that is slow growing and rarely involves the lymph nodes when the cancer is small.

tumor: a mass of abnormal cells that may be either cancerous or benign.

estrogen receptor gene: a gene associated with inhibiting the abnormal growth of cells.

unifocal: in one location.

unsaturated fat: a type of fat that may have a healthy effect on the heart when used in moderation.

vertebra: any one of the 33 bones that make up the spine.

weight-bearing exercise: exercises that put stress on muscle and bone; weight-bearing exercises help build up bone density and prevent the bones from becoming brittle.

BIBLIOGRAPHY AND FURTHER READING

Abrams J., Chen T., Giusti R. Survival after breast-sparing surgery versus mastectomy. *J Natl Cancer Inst*, 86:1672–1673, 1994.

American Joint Committee on Cancer. *AJCC Cancer Staging Manual, Fifth Edition*. Philadelphia: Lippincott-Raven, 1997.

American Society of Clinical Oncology. Recommended breast cancer surveillance guidelines: American Society of Clinical Oncology. *J Clin Oncol*, 15:2149–2156, 1997.

Anderson D. E. Familial versus sporadic breast cancer. *Cancer*, 70:1740–1746, 1992.

Assikis V. J, Neven P., Jordan V. C., et al. A realistic clinical perspective of tamoxifen and endometrial carcinogenesis. *Eur J Cancer*, 32:1464–1476, 1996.

Balducci L. Breast cancer in older women. *Am Fam Physician*, 58(5):1163–1172, 1998.

Ballo M. S., Sneige N. Can core needle biospy replace fine-needle aspiration cytology in the diagnosis of palpable breast carcinoma: a comparative study of 124 women. *Cancer*, 78:773–777, 1996.

Bartholomew L. L. The alleged association between induced abortion and risk of breast cancer: biology or bias? *Obstet Gynecol Surv*, 53(11):708–714, 1998.

Berry D. A. Benefits and risks of screening mammography for women in their forties: a statistical appraisal. *J Natl Cancer Inst* , 90(19):1431–1439, 1998.

Brenner A. J., Aldaz C. M. The genetics of sporadic breast cancer. *Prog Clin Biol Res*, 396:63–82, 1996.

Buzdar A. U. and Hortobagyi G. N. Tamoxifen and tore-mifene in breast cancer: comparison of safety and efficacy. *J Clin Oncol*, 16(1):348–353, 1998.

Cady B. Is axillary lymph node dissection necessary in routine management of breast cancer? No. *Important Adv Oncol*, 251–265, 1996.

Casey G. The BRCA1 and BRCA2 breast cancer genes. *Curr Opin Oncol*, 9:88–93, 1997.

Cheson, B. D. (editor). Thirty-fourth annual meeting highlights of the American Society of Clinical Oncology, 1998.

Chu K. C., Tarone R. E., Kessler L. G., et al. Recent trends in U.S. breast cancer incidence, survival, and mortality rates. *J Natl Cancer Inst*, 88:1571–1579, 1996.

Ciatto S., Cariaggi P., Bulgaresi P., et al. Fine needle aspiration cytology of the breast: review of 9533 consecutive cases. *Breast*, 2:87–90, 1993.

Cockburn J., Redman S., and Kricker A. Should women take part in clinical trials in breast cancer? *J Clin Oncol*, 16(1)·354–361, 1998.

Colditz G. A. Epidemiology of breast cancer: findings from the Nurses' Health Study. *Cancer*, 71:1480–1489, 1993.

Cummings S. R., Norton L., Eckert S., et al. Raloxifene reduces the risk of breast cancer and may decrease the risk of endometrial cancer in postmenopausal women: two-year findings from the Multiple Outcomes of Raloxifene Evaluation Trial. *Proc Am Soc Clin Oncol*, 17:2a, abstract, 1998.

D'Angelo P. C., Galliano D. E., Rosemurgy A. S. Stereotactic excisional breast biopsies utilizing the advanced breast biopsy instrumentation system. *Am J Surg*, 174:297–302, 1997.

DeVita V. T., Hellman S., Rosenberg S. A. (editors). *Cancer: Principles and Practice of Oncology, Fifth Edition*. Philadelphia: Lippincott-Raven, 1997.

Dewar J. A., Horobin J. M., Preece, P. E., et al. Long term effect of tamoxifen on blood lipid values in breast cancer. *BMJ*, 305:225–226, 1992.

Dickson R. B., Lippman M. E. Growth factors in breast cancer. *Endocr Rev*, 16:559–589, 1995.

Early Breast Cancer Trialists' Collaborative Group. Tamoxifen for early breast cancer: an overview of the randomised trials. *Lancet*, 351:1451–1467, 1998.

Elledge R. M., McGuire W. L., Osborne C. K. Prognostic factors in breast cancer. *Semin Oncol*, 19:244–253, 1992.

Epstein R. J. Routine or delayed axillary dissection for primary breast cancer? *Eur J Cancer*, 31A:1570–1573, 1995.

Eskelinen M. DNA flow cytometry, nuclear morphometry, mitotic indices and steroid receptors as independent prognostic factors in female breast cancer. *Int J Cancer*, 51(4):555–561, 1992.

Fisher B. Biological and clinical considerations regarding the use of surgery and chemotherapy in the treatment of primary breast cancer. *Cancer*, 40:574–587, 1997.

Fisher B., Costantino J. P., Redmond C. K., et al. Endometrial cancer in tamoxifen-treated breast cancer patients: findings from the National Surgical Adjuvant Breast and Bowel Project (NSABP) B-14. *J Natl Cancer Inst*, 86:527–537, 1994.

Fisher B., Costantino J. P., Wickerham D. L., et al. Tamoxifen for prevention of breast cancer: report of the

National Surgical Adjuvant Breast and Bowel Project P-1 Study. *J Natl Cancer Inst*, 90(18):1371–88, 1998.

Fisher B., Dignam J., Bryant J., et al. Five versus more than five years of tamoxifen therapy for breast cancer patients with negative lymph nodes and estrogen receptor negative tumors. *J Natl Cancer Inst*, 88(21):1529–1542, 1996.

Fisher B., Dignam J., Wolmark M., et al. Lumpectomy and radiation therapy for the treatment of intraductal breast cancer: findings from National Surgical Adjuvant Breast and Bowel Project B-17. *J Clin Oncol*, 16:441–452, 1998.

FitzGerald M. G., MacDonald D. J., Krainer M., et al. Germline BRCA1 mutations in Jewish and non-Jewish women with early-onset breast cancer. *N Engl J Med*, 334: 143–149, 1996.

Gams R. Phase III trials of toremifene vs tamoxifen. *Oncol*, suppl(4):23–28, 1997.

Gelber R. D., Cole B. F., Goldhirsch A., et al. Adjuvant chemotherapy plus tamoxifen compared with tamoxifen alone for postmenopausal breast cancer: Meta-analysis of quality-adjusted survival. *Lancet*, 347:1066–1071, 1996.

Ghadirian P. Sociodemographic characteristics, smoking, medical and family history, and breast cancer. *Cancer Detect Prev*, 22(6):485–494, 1998.

Gilliland F. D. Reproductive risk factors for breast cancer in Hispanic and non-Hispanic white women: the New Mexico Women's Health Study. *Am J Epidemiol*, 148(7):683–692, 1998.

Goldhirsch A. Meeting highlights: international consensus panel on the treatment of primary breast cancer. *J Natl Cancer Inst*, 90(21):1601–1608, 1998.

Goldhirsch A., Wood W. C., Senn H. J., et al. Highlights: international consensus panel on the treatment of primary breast cancer. *J Natl Cancer Inst*, 87:1441–1445, 1995.

Gradishar W. J., Jordan V. C. Clinical potential of new antiestrogens. *J Clin Oncol*, 15:840–852, 1997.

Grenman R. L., Laine K. M., Klemi P. J., et al. Effect of the antiestrogen toremifene on growth of the human mammary carcinoma cell line MCF-7. *J Cancer Res Clin Oncol*, 117:223–226, 1991.

Haffty B. G., Ward B., Pathare P., et al. Reappraisal of the role of axillary lymph node dissection in the conservative treatment of breast cancer. *J Clin Oncol*, 15:691–700, 1997.

Hall F. M. Technologic advances in breast imaging: current and future strategies, controversies, and opportunities. *Surg Oncol Clin North Am*, 6:403–409, 1997.

Hayes D. F., Van Zyl J. A., Hacking A., et al. Randomized comparison of tamoxifen and two separate doses of toremifene in postmenopausal patients with metastatic breast cancer. *J Clin Oncol*, 13(10):2556–2566, 1995.

Hortobagyi G. N. Treatment of breast cancer. *N Engl J Med*, 339(14):974–982, 1998.

Hoskins K. F., Stopfer J. E., Calzone K. A., et al. Assessment and counseling for women with a family history of breast cancer: a guide for clinicians. *JAMA*, 273:577–585, 1995.

Jaiyesimi I. A., Buzdar A. U., Hortobagyi G. N. Inflammatory breast cancer: a review. *J Clin Oncol*, 10:1014–1024, 1992.

Jordan V. A., Morrow M. Should clinicians be concerned about the carcinogenic potential of tamoxifen? *Eur J Cancer*, 30:1724–1721, 1994.

Jordan V. C., Gradishar W. J. Molecular mechanisms and future uses of antiestrogens. *Mol Aspects Med*, 18:171–224, 1997.

Kerlikowske K., Grady D., Rubin S. M., et al. Efficacy of screening mammography: a meta-analysis. *JAMA*, 273:149–154, 1998.

Khalkhali I., Mena I., Diggles L. Review of imaging techniques for the diagnosis of breast cancer: a new role of prone scintimammography using technetium-99m sestamibi. *Eur J Nuc Med*, 21:357–362, 1994.

Kollias J. Screening women aged less than 50 years with a family history of breast cancer. *Eur J Cancer*, 34(6): 878–883, 1998.

Krag D., Weaver D., Ashikaga T., et al. The sentinel node in breast cancer: a multicenter validation study. *N Engl J Med*, 339(14):941–946, 1998.

Kuss J., Muss S. B., Hoen H., et al. Tamoxifen as initial endocrine therapy for metastatic breast cancer: long term follow-up of two Piedmont Oncology Association (POA) trials. *Breast Cancer Res Treat*, 42:265–274, 1997.

Lalloo F. Screening by mammography, women with a family history of breast cancer. *Eur J Cancer*, 34(6):937–940, 1998.

Leitch A. M., Dodd G. D., Costanza M., et al. American Cancer Society guidelines for the early detection of breast cancer: update 1997. *CA Cancer J Clin*, 47:150–153, 1997.

Levine M. N., Gent M., Hirsh J., et al. The thrombogenic effect of anticancer drug therapy in women with stage II breast cancer. *N Engl J Med*, 318:404–407, 1988.

Love R. R., Mazess R. B., Barden H. S., et al. Effects of tamoxifen on bone mineral density in postmenopausal women with breast cancer. *N Engl J Med*, 326:852–856, 1992.

Love R. R., Newcomb P. A., Wiebe D. A., et al. Lipid and lipoprotein effects of tamoxifen therapy in postmenopausal patients with node negative breast cancer. *J Natl Cancer Inst*, 82:1322–1327, 1990.

Madigan M. P., Ziegler R. G., Benichou J., et al. Proportion of breast cancer cases in the United States explained by well-established risk factors. *J Natl Cancer Inst*, 87:1681–1685, 1995.

Magriples U, Naftolin F, Schwartz P. E., et al. High grade endometrial carcinoma in tamoxifen-treated breast cancer patients. *J Clin Oncol*, 11:485–490, 1993.

Malkin D., Li F. P., Strong L. C., et al. Germ line p53 mutations in a familial syndrome of breast cancer, sarcomas, and other neoplasms. *Science*, 250: 1233–1238, 1990.

Mansour E. G. The value of prognostic factors in selecting node-negative breast cancer patients for adjuvant therapy. *J Surg Oncol*, 49(2):73–75, 1992.

Marcus J. N., Watson P., Page D. L., et al. Hereditary breast cancer: pathobiology, prognosis, and BRCA1 and BRCA2 gene linkage. *Cancer*, 77:697–709, 1996.

McDonald C. C., Alexander F. E., Whyte B. W., et al. Cardiac and vascular morbidity in women receiving adjuvant tamoxifen for breast cancer in a randomized trial. The Scottish Cancer Trials Breast Group. *BMJ*, 311:977–980, 1995.

McGuire W. L. Prognostic factors and treatment decisions in axillary-node-negative breast cancer. *N Engl J Med*, 326(26):1756–1761, 1992.

McKenzie K., Sukumar S. Molecular genetics of human breast cancer. *Prog Clin Biol Res*, 394:183–209, 1996.

McMasters K. M., Giuliano A. E., Ross M. I., et al. Sentinel-lymph-node biopsy for breast cancer—not yet the standard of care. *N Engl J Med*, 339(14):990–995, 1998.

Morris A. D., Morris R. D., Wilson J. F., et al. Breast-conserving therapy vs mastectomy in early-stage breast cancer: a meta-analysis of 10-year survival. *Cancer J Sci Am*, 3:6–12, 1997.

Murphy B., Muss H. B. Hormonal therapy of breast cancer: state of the art. *Oncology*, suppl(4):7–18, 1997.

Muss H. B. Endocrine therapy for advanced breast cancer: a review. *Breast Cancer Res Treat*, 21:15–26, 1992.

National Cancer Institute. SEER Cancer Statistics Review 1973-1990, Document 93-2789. Bethesda, MD, NCI, 1993.

Nayfield S. G., Gorin M. B. Tamoxifen-associated eye disease: a review. *J Clin Oncol*, 14:1018–1026, 1996.

Osborne C. K. Prognostic factors for breast cancer: have they met their promise? *J Clin Oncol*, 10(5):679–682, 1992.

Ozer H. (editor). Selected highlights of reports at the 34th annual meeting of the American Society of Clinical Oncology, 1998.

Page D. L., Dupont W. D. Premalignant conditions and markers of elevated risk in the breast and their management. *Surg Clin North Am*, 70:831–851, 1990.

Parker S. L., Tong T., Bolden S., et al. Cancer statistics, 1997. *CA Cancer J Clin*, 47:5–27, 1997.

Perry M. C. (editor). *Controversies in the management of early-stage breast cancer.* American Society of Clinical Oncology Educational Book, 34th Annual Meeting, 1998.

Perry M. C. (editor). *How to break bad news to patients with cancer.* American Society of Clinical Oncology Educational Book, 34th Annual Meeting, 1998.

Perry M. C. (editor). *Implications of genetic testing for practicing physicians.* American Society of Clinical Oncology Edu-cational Book, 34th Annual Meeting, 1998.

Perry M. C. (editor). *Inherited breast cancer susceptibility and testing prevention.* American Society of Clinical Oncology Educational Book, 34th Annual Meeting, 1998.

Powles T., Eeles R., Ashly S., et al. Interim analysis of the incidence of breast cancer in the Royal Marsden Hospital tamoxifen randomised chemoprevention trial. *Lancet*, 352(9122):98–101, 1998.

Pritchard K. I. Is tamoxifen effective in prevention of breast cancer? (editorial). *Lancet*, 352(9122):80–81, 1998.

Ragaz J, Jackson S. M., Le N., et al. Adjuvant radiotherapy and chemotherapy in node-positive premenopausal women with breast cancer. *N Engl J Med*, 337:956–962, 1997.

Rakowsky E. Prognostic factors in node-positive operable breast cancer patients receiving adjuvant chemotherapy. *Breast Cancer Res Treat*, 21(2):121–131, 1992.

Robinson E., Kimmick G. G., Muss H. B. Tamoxifen in postmenopausal women: A safety perspective. *Drugs Aging*, 8:329–337, 1996.

Rockhill B. Age at menarche, time to regular cycling, and breast cancer. *Cancer Causes Control*, 9(4):447–453, 1998.

Rosenberg K. Ten-year risk of false positive screening mammograms and clinical breast examinations. *J Nurse Midwifery*, 43(5):394–395, 1998.

Rutqvist L. E., Mattsson A. Cardiac and thromboembolic morbidity among postmenopausal women with early-stage breast cancer in a randomized trial of adjuvant tamoxifen. The Stockholm Breast Cancer Study Group. *J Natl Cancer Inst*, 85:1398–1406, 1993.

Sacks F. M., Walsh B. W. Sex hormones and lipoprotein metabolism. *Curr Opin Lipidol*, 5:236–240, 1994.

Schlesinger C. Endometrial polyps: a comparison study of patients receiving tamoxifen with two control groups. *Int J Gynecol Pathol*, 17(4):302–311, 1998.

Schwartzberg L. S. Sequential treatment including high-dose chemotherapy with peripheral blood stem cell support in patients with high-risk stage II-III breast cancer: outpatient administration in community cancer centers. *Am J Clin Oncol*, 21(5):523–531, 1998.

Shewmon D. A., Stock J. L., Rosen C. J., et al. Tamoxifen and estrogen lower circulating lipoprotein (a) concentrations in healthy postmenopausal women. *Arterioscler Thromb*, 14:1586–1593, 1994.

Slamon D. J., Clark G. M., Wong S. G., et al. Human breast cancer: correlation of relapse and survival with amplification of the HER2/neu oncogene. *Science*, 235:177–182, 1987.

Solin L. J., Kurtz J., Fourquet A., et al. Fifteen-year results of breast-conserving surgery and definitive breast irradiation for the treatment of ductal carcinoma in situ of the breast. *J Clin Oncol*, 14:754–763, 1996.

Stenbygaard L. E., Herrstedt J., Thomsen J. F., et al. Toremifene and tamoxifen in advanced breast cancer—a double-blind crossover trial. *Breast Cancer Res Treat*, 25:57–63, 1993.

Swedish Breast Cancer Cooperative Group. Randomized trial of two versus five years of adjuvant tamoxifen for postmenopausal early stage breast cancer. *J Natl Cancer Inst*, 88:1543–1549, 1996.

Szamel I., Vincze B., Hindy I., et al. Hormonal effects of toremifene in breast cancer patients. *J Steroid Biochem*, 136:243–247, 1990.

The GIVIO investigators. Impact of follow-up testing on survival and health-related quality of life in breast cancer patients: a multicenter randomized clinical trial. *JAMA*, 271:1587–1592, 1994.

Tomas E., Kauppila A., Blanco G., et al. Comparison between the effects of tamoxifen and toremifene on the uterus in postmenopausal breast cancer patients. *Gynecol Oncol*, 59:261–266, 1995.

Tormey D. C., Gray R., Falkson H. C. Postchemotherapy adjuvant tamoxifen therapy beyond 5 years in patients with lymph node positive breast cancer. *J Natl Cancer Inst*, 88:1828–1833, 1996.

Troisi R. Pregnancy characteristics and maternal risk of breast cancer. *Epidemiology*, 9(6):641–647, 1998.

Veronesi U., Maisonneuve P., Costa A., et al. Prevention of breast cancer with tamoxifen: preliminary findings from the

Italian randomised trial among hysterectomised women. *Lancet*, 352(9122):93–97, 1998.

Veronesi U., Paganelli G., Galimberti V., et al. Sentinel-node biopsy to avoid axillary dissection in breast cancer with clinically negative lymph-nodes. *Lancet*, 349:1864–1867, 1997.

Veronesi U., Salvadori B., Luini A., et al. Conservative treatment of early breast cancer. Long-term results of 1232 cases treated with quadrantectomy, axillary dissection, and radiotherapy. *Ann Surg*, 211:250–259, 1990.

Von Kleist, S. Prognostic factors in breast cancer: theoretical and clinical aspects (review). *Anticancer Res*, 16(6C):3907–3912, 1996.

Wakeling A. E. The future of new pure antiestrogens in clinical breast cancer. *Breast Cancer Res Treat*, 25:1–9, 1993.

Warri A. M., Huovinon R. L., Laine A. M., et al. Apoptosis in toremifene growth inhibition of human breast cancer cells in vivo and in vitro. *J Natl Cancer Inst*, 85:1412–1418, 1993.

White R. R. Incidence of breast carcinoma in patients having reduction mammaplasty. *Plast Reconstr Surg*, 102(5): 1774–1775, 1998.

Yao K., Jordan V. C. Questions about tamoxifen and the future use of antiestrogens. *The Oncologist*, 3:104–110, 1998.

Yu H. Alcohol consumption and breast cancer risk. *JAMA*, 280(13):1138–1139, 1998.

Zedeler K., Keiding N., Kamby C. Differential influence of prognostic factors on the occurrence of metastases at various anatomical sites in human breast cancer. *Stat Med*, 11(3):281–294, 1992.

Zeneca Pharmaceuticals. Full prescribing information, 1998.

Zeneca Pharmaceuticals. Nolvadex, clinical management of breast cancer: insights on current practices for adjuvant therapy, 1996.

INDEX

Abortion, risk of breast cancer and, 30
Adjuvant therapy with tamoxifen, 103–22
  benefits of, 110–13
  case study in, 103–5
  chemotherapy vs., 107–9
  clinical studies of, 113–17
  deciding whether to use, 106–7
  effectiveness of, 89–90, 93
  for estrogen receptor negative cancer, 115, 117
  for estrogen receptor positive cancer, 114–15
  for metastatic breast cancer, 117–22
  purpose of, 88–89, 105–6
  risk reduction with, 89–90, 114–17
Age factors
  in Breast Cancer Risk Assessment Tool, 135
  breast cancer survival and, 10
  candidacy for tamoxifen therapy and, 138–39
  mammography screening and, 35, 37
  risk of breast cancer and, 24–25
Alcohol, risk of breast cancer and, 33
Alternative therapy, resources for, 168
Androgen therapy, for metastatic breast cancer, 121
Antiestrogens, 152–53
Aromatase inhibitors, for metastatic breast cancer, 120
Axillary lymph node dissection
  for evaluation of metastasis, 73–74
  during lumpectomy, 67–68
  lymphedema related to, 74
  sentinel node biopsy vs., 74–75
Axillary lymph nodes, 8

Biomarkers, 58–59
Biopsy
  core needle, 52–53
  excisional, 55–57
  fine needle aspiration, 49–52
  incisional, 54–55
  second opinion for, 53
  of sentinel node, 74–75
  types of, 54
  wire localization in, 56
Biopsy gun, 52
Blood clots, 99, 134

Bone marrow transplantation, after high-dose chemotherapy, 111
Bones. *See also* Osteoporosis
  pain in, as reaction to tamoxifen therapy, 121
  tamoxifen effects in, 96
BRCA1 and BRCA2 genes, 26–27, 129
Breast
  anatomy of, 4–8
  disorders of, 18–19, 31
  hormonal effects on, 8–9, 29–31
  milk production and delivery system in, 5–7
  rare, benign conditions of, 19
  tamoxifen effects in, 96
Breast cancer. *See also* Metastatic breast cancer
  books about, 168–72
  breast anatomy and, 4–8
  case study in, 1–2
  characteristics of women with (epidemiology), 10–11
  in contralateral breast, prevention by tamoxifen, 112, 116
  diagnosis and screening of. *See* Diagnosis and screening
  ductal carcinoma in situ, 12–14, 16, 53, 128
  estrogen receptor negative cancer, 89–90, 103, 114–15
  estrogen receptor positive, 90, 95–96, 115, 117
  genetic factors in, 9–10, 22–23, 25–26
  incidence of, 3, 11
  invasive types of, 15–16
  lobular carcinoma in situ, 5–6, 14–16, 135, 127–29
  prognosis in, 17–18, 76
  rare types of, 16–17
  recurrence of, tamoxifen prevention of, 114–16
  reduction of risk for. *See* Risk reduction, with tamoxifen
  risk factors for. *See* Risk factors for breast cancer
  surgery for. *See* Surgery
  survival and mortality in, 3–4, 10, 17, 115–17
  symptoms of, 11–12
  in younger women, 10

198